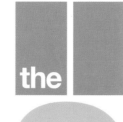

the 2 day diet cookbook

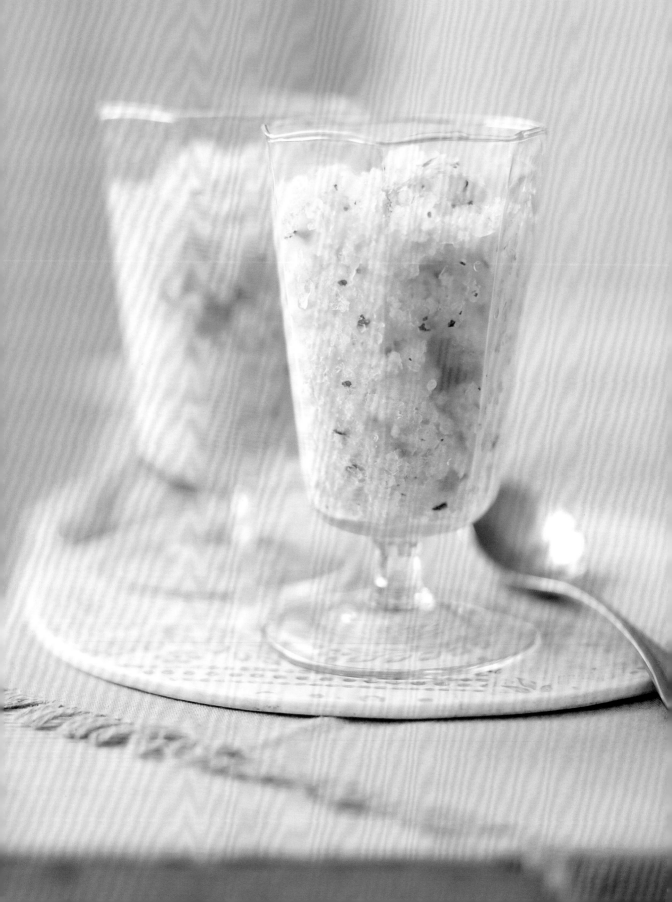

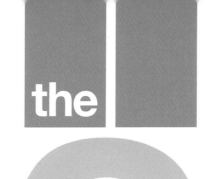

the 2 day diet cookbook

Diet two days a week.
Eat normally for five.

Dr Michelle Harvie & Prof Tony Howell

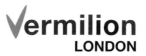

Vermilion
LONDON

This book is dedicated to the numerous dieters who have taken part in our 2-Day Diet research, which has informed this ground-breaking Diet. Thanks to them, we know that The 2-Day Diet works and has numerous health benefits. Our dieters have provided invaluable insights and tips concerning what really helps them keep to the Diet.

10 9 8 7 6 5 4

Published in 2013 by Vermilion, an imprint of Ebury Publishing
A Random House Group company

Recipes by Emily Jonzen
Photography by Ian Greig Garlick

The Random House Group Limited Reg. No. 954009

Addresses for companies within the Random House Group can be found at www.randomhouse.co.uk

The Random House Group Limited supports the Forest Stewardship Council® (FSC®), the leading international forest-certification organisation. Our books carrying the FSC label are printed on FSC®-certified paper. FSC is the only forest-certification scheme supported by the leading environmental organisations, including Greenpeace. Our paper procurement policy can be found at www.randomhouse.co.uk/environment

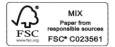

Produced by Bookworx
Project editor: Jo Godfrey Wood
Project designer: Peggy Sadler

Home economist: Emma Marsden

Printed and bound in the UK by Butler Tanner and Dennis Ltd

ISBN 978-0-09-195468-0

To buy books by your favourite authors and register for offers visit www.randomhouse.co.uk

All author proceeds from the sale of this book will go to Genesis Breast Cancer Prevention (Registered Charity Number 1109839).

genesis   www.genesisuk.org

The information in this book has been compiled by way of general guidance in relation to the specific subjects addressed, but is not a substitute and not to be relied on for medical, healthcare, pharmaceutical or other professional advice on specific circumstances and in specific locations. Please consult your GP before changing, stopping or starting any medical treatment. So far as the author is aware the information given is correct and up to date as at April 2013. Practice, laws and regulations all change and the reader should obtain up-to-date professional advice on any such issues. The author and publishers disclaim, as far as the law allows, any liability arising directly or indirectly from the use, or misuse, of the information contained in this book.

contents

introduction

The right diet for you

If you are searching for a safe and rigorously tested diet, one that really does help you to lose weight and keep it off, The 2-Day Diet is a brand-new approach that has proven results. Not only will it enable you to lose weight and keep it off, but it will also help to protect you against cancer and improve your health generally. The 2-Day Diet is associated with lowering high blood pressure and anti-ageing effects, as well as with improving general well-being, mood and energy levels. It will also help to retrain your appetite so that you can move away from over-eating and unhealthy food cravings. In short, it will help you learn to eat what your body actually wants and needs, so that you lose weight and keep it off.

To experience all the benefits of The 2-Day Diet you don't have to fast, skip meals or feel hungry. All you need to do is eat a low-carbohydrate, high protein diet for two days a week, ideally consecutively, and then eat normally but sensibly for the other five days.

IF YOU ARE VEGETARIAN

You can follow The 2-Day Diet if you are vegetarian. Just be sure you eat enough protein to help you feel full.

This book includes vegetarian recipes and plenty of ideas to adapt the other recipes for vegetarians. The information on following the vegetarian version of the Diet is on pages 142–5.

Rapid results

We developed the The 2-Day Diet with short- and long-term weight loss in mind: you can expect to see rapid results – up to 2 kg (4 lb 4 oz) of fat lost a week. In clinical trials, 2-Day Dieters lost fat about one and a half times more quickly than those on a conventional seven-day, calorie-controlled diet and lost more centimetres around their waists, which is where fat most harmful to your health is stored. After a month on the Diet we found that 2-Day Dieters lost on average 0.5–1.4 kg (1–3 lb) a week, whereas 7-day dieters only lost an average of 0.3–1 kg (½–2 lb) a week.

Longer term, our 2-Day Dieters were also more successful in keeping the weight off. In one study 70 per cent of the 2-Day Dieters were still following the Diet after three months, compared with only 40 per cent of the 7-day dieters. In another, we followed 2-Day Dieters for 12–15 months after they first started the Diet and found that they kept their weight off and maintained healthier lower levels of cholesterol and the hormone insulin with one restricted day per week. You can read in detail how we developed the Diet over the last 12 years and find out about the clinical trials we carried out in our first book, *The 2-Day Diet*.

Easy to fit into daily and family life

The 2-Day Diet is not only easy to stick to but it's also easy to fit around your daily life. On your restricted, low-carb days you can still eat the same as your family or partner, but simply add portions of carbohydrate foods, such as

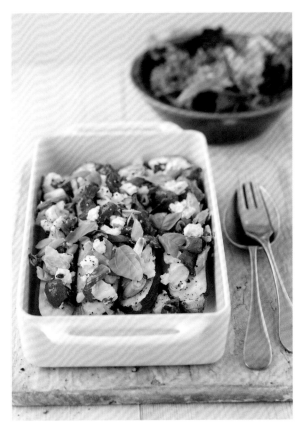
Stuffed courgettes with feta and sundried tomatoes, page 84.

THE 2-DAY DIET IN FIVE EASY STEPS

1 On The 2-Day Diet you eat a low-carb diet for two days a week and normally but sensibly for the other five.

2 Look up how many servings of protein, dairy, fats, vegetables and carbohydrates you can eat per day on your restricted and unrestricted days in the Ready Reckoner charts on pages 146-9.

3 Consult the lists of foods on pages 142–5 to find out what a serving looks like.

4 Plan what to eat each week. To help you get started there are meal planners on pages 150–3 and a list of the recipes on pages 140–1.

5 Get cooking, enjoy great healthy food and start losing weight!

rice, pasta or baked potatoes, to their meals. The healthy meals designed for the other five days of the week are ideal for the whole family. Everyone will thoroughly enjoy the meals in this book and none of you should feel as though you are 'on a diet'.

Are you overweight?

You probably know if you are overweight, but it will help you plan your weight loss and establish your goal weight if you know how much you weigh. Start by weighing yourself and then go to our website www.thetwodaydiet.co.uk to work out your body mass index (BMI). Although your BMI doesn't give the whole story, a healthy BMI is in the region of 18.5–24.9. If yours is higher

than this, you need to think about losing weight. If you are very overweight, start by setting yourself a shorter-term goal rather than one that seems unattainable. For more information about what is a healthy weight and setting weight-loss goals see *The 2-Day Diet*.

How to do The 2-Day Diet

The 2-Day Diet includes a low-carbohydrate diet for two days a week. These are your 'restricted' days and it is best if you run these two days back to back. Although you can lose weight if you space them out over the week, our trials showed that Dieters found the second day as easy as, or easier than, the first when they did them together because they had got into the

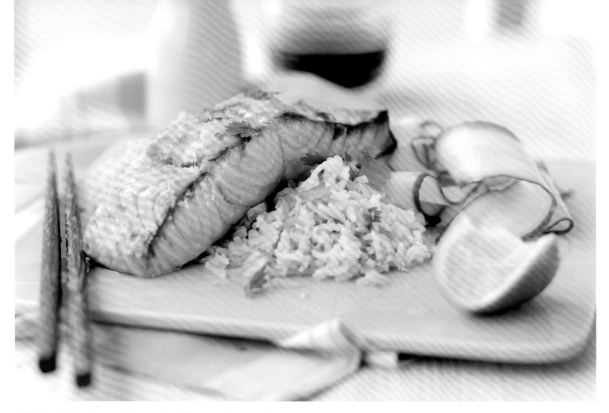

Grilled teriyaki salmon with cucumber ribbons and sesame rice, page 116.

habit of eating less. There is also evidence that there are additional health benefits from doing the two days together because the body is in a healthier metabolic state for a longer period.

On your restricted days you eat lots of protein, healthy fats, low-fat dairy foods and some vegetables and fruit. You need to restrict your intake of carbohydrate to around 50 g (2 oz) per day, which is why you avoid all foods such as rice and pasta and also higher-carbohydrate fruit and vegetables, such as carrots, blueberries and onions. These higher-carbohydrate fruit and vegetables are, of course, still healthy foods and you can eat these on your unrestricted days.

The Diet is extremely simple to follow. There is no calorie-counting and no need for vitamin supplements. You are advised to eat the recommended number of servings from different food groups (i.e. protein, fat, dairy or vegetables).

YOUR DAILY ALLOWANCE ON EACH OF THE 2 RESTRICTED DAYS

For serving sizes see pages 142–5

Protein 4–12 servings for women and 4–14 for men of: fish, seafood, skinless chicken and turkey, lean beef, pork, lamb or offal, eggs, tofu, Quorn, TVP, tempeh or soya beans

Fats Up to 5 servings for women and up to 6 for men of: healthy fats such as olive oil, nuts and peanut butter

Dairy 3 servings of semi-skimmed milk, low-fat yoghurt or reduced-fat cheese

Vegetables/salad 5 servings of low-carb vegetables, such as green veg

Fruit 1 piece of low-carb fruit

Drinks at least 2 litres (3½ pints) of water, tea, coffee or low-cal drinks

The box below left shows how many servings of a particular food group you can eat per day on each of your two restricted days. These are the maximum amounts and you don't have to eat all of your allowance if you feel full. Do, however, try to eat the minimum amount of protein and all of your dairy, fruit and vegetable allowance and to drink plenty of the permitted drinks. Tables at the back of the book on pages 142–5 explain what a serving of food looks like.

What to eat for the rest of the week

For the remainder of the week, on your unrestricted days, we recommend that you eat normally but sensibly. The two restricted days help retrain your appetite so that you won't want to eat as much as you might normally. Listen to how hungry you feel and don't just eat the same amount as you would usually, out of habit. Most of us actually eat more than our body needs.

We have provided diet Ready Reckoners on pages 146–9 to help you work out how much you should actually be eating on your unrestricted days, based on your age, gender and current weight. We recommend a healthy diet with plenty of fresh fish, lean meat, salad, vegetables, fruit and wholegrains. On unrestricted days you can eat all types of vegetables, fruits and salads – so if the one you want is not listed in the tables, work out what a serving size might look like from a similar food listed in that food group.

Try to avoid ready meals and processed foods as these are often high in sugar and fat, and can be less satisfying. If you are someone who cannot imagine a week without a glass of wine or beer or unhealthy foods, such as biscuits or crisps, you can still have these. However,

ABOUT THE READY RECKONERS

Use the Ready Reckoner charts on pages 146–9 to find out how many servings of food you can have per day, according to your gender, age and current weight. They include information for weight loss and maintenance.

• It is important to get enough protein, dairy, fruit and vegetables on the 2 restricted and 5 unrestricted days. This is why you need to eat the minimum recommended protein allowance and your dairy, fruit and vegetable allowance each day. These Ready Reckoners have been designed so that you will achieve the recommended amount of 1.2 g of protein per kg of body weight per day.

• You do not need to eat the maximum amounts on the table. However, it is important to get the balance of foods right. For example, if you only have two-thirds of your maximum protein servings you should also roughly aim for two-thirds of your maximum fat and high-fibre carbohydrate servings.

to get the full benefit of this diet we strongly recommend that you restrict alcohol to no more than ten units a week and only have three servings of less healthy 'treat' foods a week. We have given some examples of treat servings and a guide to alcohol servings on page 145.

To help you get started on the Diet we have provided three weeks of meal plans for both non-vegetarians (see pages 150–1) and vegetarians (see pages 152–3). These will give you a feel for what and how much to eat on the restricted and unrestricted days.

A NOTE ABOUT THE RECIPES

- Most of the recipes serve one, two or four people. If you are increasing quantities to feed more people, you may also need to adjust the cooking times.
- All spoon measurements are level, unless otherwise indicated, and are assumed to be standard sizes: teaspoon = 5 ml, tablespoon = 15 ml. If you are in any doubt, buy a set of spoon measures.
- All hobs and ovens differ, so check as you cook. The oven temperatures given are for conventional electric ovens and gas ovens; for fan-assisted ovens, subtract 20°C from the suggested cooking temperature.
- All eggs are 'medium', ideally free-range.

Each recipe shows how many servings it contributes to your allowance in The 2-Day Diet plan. Many foods contain a combination of nutrients, some of which are in such small quantities they do not count towards your serving allowances. All servings have been rounded to the nearest half.

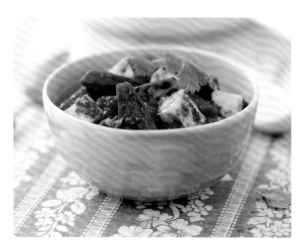

Okra and tomato curry with paneer, page 80.

There are also 65 recipes in this book, many of them illustrated, to help you eat well every day and really enjoy your food on this diet. We want The 2-Day Diet to work for you, so that you learn to love real food, improve your health and help protect yourself against disease. The 2-Day Diet should become a way of life rather than a short-term fix that will help you lose weight now, only to pile it back on later.

How to get maximum benefit from the Diet

To boost weight loss and the health benefits of the Diet we recommend that you become more active. The 2-Day Diet is good at targeting fat and preserving muscle during weight loss, but this will be further boosted with exercise. Exercise also helps you to feel more energetic and can help improve your mood as well. You can exercise on both your restricted and unrestricted days. If you are someone who never exercises, just start by becoming more active and walking more. Aim to build up to 150 minutes of being active a week – everything counts, including going up and down the stairs or walking vigorously to the bus stop. For detailed advice on exercise please refer to *The 2-Day Diet* book and website (www. thetwodaydiet.co.uk).

How do I keep off the weight I've lost?

Once you have reached your goal weight you can keep the weight off by doing just one restricted day per week. This will also help maintain the health benefits of the Diet, including lower levels of insulin and other hormones, which are the cause of many diseases, such as cancer and diabetes. Continue to weigh yourself once a week to keep an eye on your weight. If you notice it creeping up more

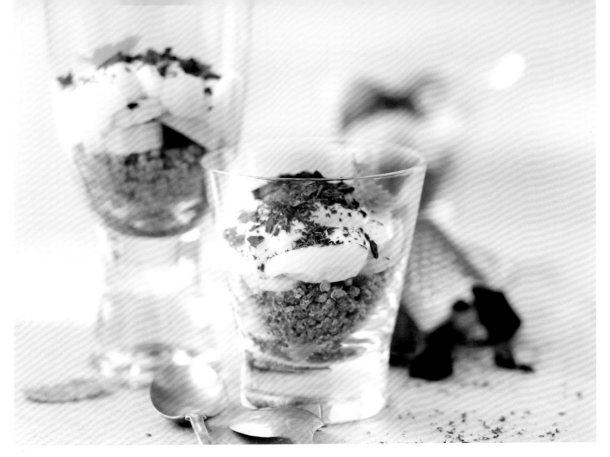

Mini banoffee pies, page 134.

than 2 kg (4 lb) we recommend going back to doing two restricted days a week until you get back to your goal weight. This will help ensure that you stay trim and healthy in the long term.

Our research at Genesis Breast Cancer Prevention is dedicated to preventing breast cancer and losing just 5 to 10 per cent of your body weight and keeping it off (if you are overweight) can reduce your risk of developing cancer and many other life-threatening diseases such as heart disease, diabetes and high blood pressure by 25 to 60 per cent. We hope that The 2-Day Diet can help you not just lose weight and feel better but also help to protect your health in the short- and long-term, so that you can lead a full, active and happy life.

Dr Michelle Harvie and Professor Tony Howell

part 1 restricted days

recipes

V indicates that the recipe is suitable for vegetarians; VT indicates vegetarian tip – that the recipe includes advice on adapting it for vegetarians.

ALL ABOUT SALT

Because you are fat-burning and passing water and electrolytes on your restricted days, you must drink plenty (2 litres/3½ pints) and include some salt, but you don't need huge amounts. If you find you are developing headaches on your restricted days, this may indicate that you need a little more water and salt.

There is some salt naturally occurring in some of the foods you will eat – for example dairy foods, fish and seafood. If you wish, you can include 4–6 servings of foods that are higher in salt on your restricted days. These foods are indicated in the serving sizes lists on pages 142–3 with *. Alternatively, you can include one serving of the following:

- ½ stock cube or 2 teaspoons bouillon as a drink or in food
- 1 tablespoon soy sauce
- 1 teaspoon yeast extract or meat stock with hot water
- 3 teaspoons gravy powder or granules dissolved in hot water

Do not include a salty drink or salty foods if you are taking a water tablet for high blood pressure.

Since too much salt is bad for blood pressure and bones we recommend that you limit these salty foods during the rest of the week to just one serving per week.

SNACK IDEAS/THE 2 RESTRICTED DAYS

- olives
- handful of any nuts (except chestnuts)
- low-carb fruit from the allowed list
- low-carb vegetable crudités such as celery, cucumber, green peppers, mangetout, spring onions and cherry tomatoes – with salsa, low-fat hummus, tsatsiki or guacamole
- yoghurt
- bowl of soup
- salad or cooked vegetables with cottage cheese, low-fat cream cheese or hummus
- half a pot of cottage cheese
- smoothie made with yoghurt, skimmed or semi-skimmed milk and one piece of fruit
- half a tin of sardines or pilchards
- sautéed tofu or chicken strips lightly fried in spices and sesame seeds
- boiled egg
- avocado, mozzarella, tomato and basil skewers or stacks
- celery sticks filled with low-fat cream cheese or peanut butter
- asparagus spears dipped in boiled egg
- sugar-free jelly
- ice lolly made from frozen, diluted, sugar-free fruit cordial

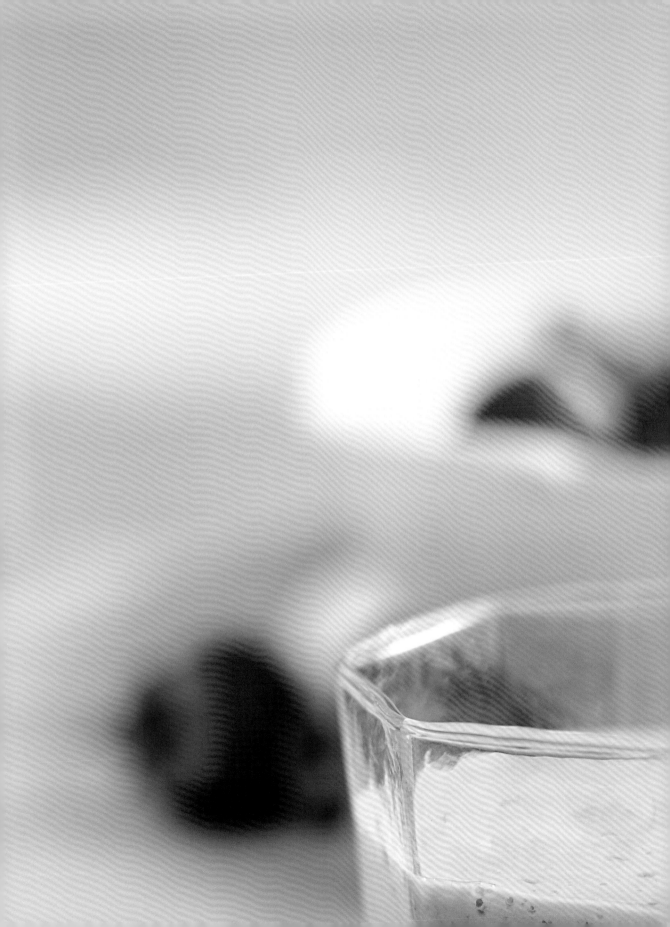

restricted days
breakfasts

boiled eggs with asparagus & ham soldiers

Use crisp, ham-wrapped asparagus instead of stodgy bread for dipping into boiled eggs.

Ingredients

2 eggs

4 slices ham, wafer-thin

80 g (2¾ oz) asparagus spears

½ tsp chives

Method

1 Carefully place the eggs in a pan of boiling water and allow to simmer for 4 minutes for soft-boiled. Remove from the water and set aside.

2 Meanwhile, cut each slice of ham in half and wrap 1 or 2 pieces around each asparagus spear, until all the slices are used up.

3 Place the wrapped spears, seam-side down, under a medium–hot grill for 3–4 minutes, until the asparagus is slightly tender and the ham is crisp.

4 Once the eggs have cooled to the touch, cut the tops off, sprinkle with the chives and use the asparagus soldiers to dip in to the yolk.

Tips & variations

If you'd like a spicy kick, try sprinkling a pinch of cayenne pepper over the soft yolks when you cut the eggs open. For a vegetarian option, leave out the ham.

SERVINGS		NUTRITION	
0	Carbohydrates	231	Calories
3	Protein	2 g	Carbohydrates
0	Fat	23 g	Protein
0	Dairy	2 g	Fibre
1	Vegetables	1.3 g	Salt
0	Fruit		

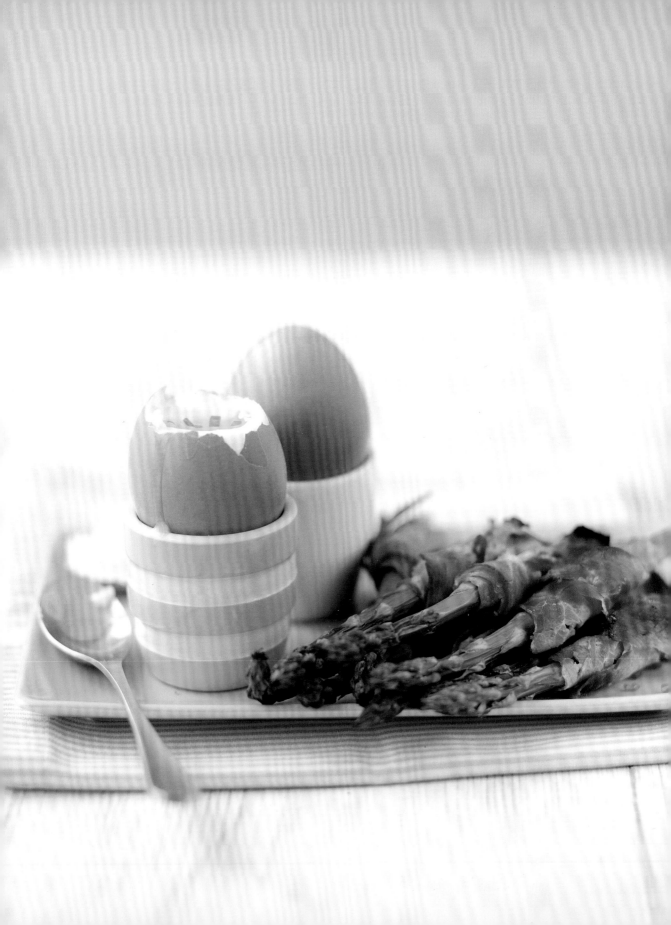

skinny English breakfast

This light version of a full English breakfast will set you up perfectly for your busy day.

Ingredients

1 clove garlic, crushed

1 tsp rapeseed oil

7 cherry tomatoes

80 g (2¾ oz) chestnut mushrooms, roughly sliced

2 rashers lean, unsmoked back bacon

1 egg

black pepper

Method

1 Preheat the grill to medium–high heat. Mix together the garlic and oil and season with a little black pepper.

2 Tip the tomatoes and mushrooms into the bowl and toss them to coat thoroughly with the garlic oil.

3 Place the tomatoes, mushrooms and bacon on a grill pan and grill for 5–6 minutes, turning everything over halfway through cooking.

4 Meanwhile bring a pan of water to the boil. Create a whirlpool by stirring with a wooden spoon and crack the egg into the middle of it.

5 Turn the heat down and simmer for 4 minutes. Drain well and serve with the bacon, mushrooms and tomatoes.

Tips & variations

You can replace the cherry tomatoes with a medium-sized tomato sliced in half. For a vegetarian option, use a vegetarian sausage instead of the bacon.

SERVINGS		NUTRITION	
0	Carbohydrates	282	Calories
3	Protein	5 g	Carbohydrates
½	Fat	26 g	Protein
0	Dairy	2 g	Fibre
2	Vegetables	3.2 g	Salt
0	Fruit		

spiced tofu scramble

This spicy breakfast makes an interesting alternative to normal scrambled eggs.

Ingredients

½ tsp olive oil

¼ tsp ground cumin

¼ tsp ground coriander

chilli flakes, pinch

100 g (3½ oz) extra-firm tofu, drained and crumbled

40 g (1½ oz) button mushrooms, halved

40 g (1½ oz) baby leaf spinach

2 spring onions, finely sliced

1 tsp flat-leaf parsley, roughly chopped

1 tsp tarragon, roughly chopped

black pepper

Method

1 Heat the oil in a frying pan over a medium heat. When hot, add the spices and chilli flakes and cook, stirring, for 30 seconds.

2 Add the tofu and mushrooms and cook for a further 2 minutes, until the mushrooms are golden.

3 Lower the heat, add the spinach and cook, stirring, for 1 minute, until the spinach has wilted.

4 Season with black pepper and serve sprinkled with the spring onions and herbs.

Tips & variations

You can also make this recipe with 2 eggs instead of the tofu.

SERVINGS	
0	Carbohydrates
2	Protein
0	Fat
0	Dairy
1	Vegetables
0	Fruit

NUTRITION	
111	Calories
2 g	Carbohydrates
10 g	Protein
3 g	Fibre
0.2 g	Salt

grilled kipper with poached egg

This satisfying breakfast provides the perfect nutrients for one of your restricted days.

Ingredients

1 egg

80 g (2¾ oz) spring greens, finely sliced

90 g (3 oz) kipper fillet, bones removed

1 tsp chives, roughly chopped

black pepper

Method

1 Preheat the grill to medium–high heat. Bring a pan of water to the boil, create a whirlpool by stirring with a wooden spoon and crack the egg into the middle of it.

2 Turn the heat down and simmer for 4 minutes. In the last minute of cooking time, place a steamer basket (or small colander) containing the spring greens over the pan.

3 Drain the egg and greens well. Meanwhile, grill the kipper for 3–4 minutes, until it is golden and piping hot.

4 Serve the kipper on a bed of spring greens, topped with the poached egg, scattered with chives and black pepper.

Tips & variations

For an easy alternative to a poached egg, boil the egg for 6 minutes before peeling and cutting it in half and serving it with the kipper. If you are vegetarian you can make this recipe with 2 poached eggs instead of the kipper fillet (to give you 2 servings of protein).

SERVINGS		NUTRITION	
0	Carbohydrates	261	Calories
4	Protein	3 g	Carbohydrates
0	Fat	22 g	Protein
0	Dairy	2 g	Fibre
1	Vegetables	1.6 g	Salt
0	Fruit		

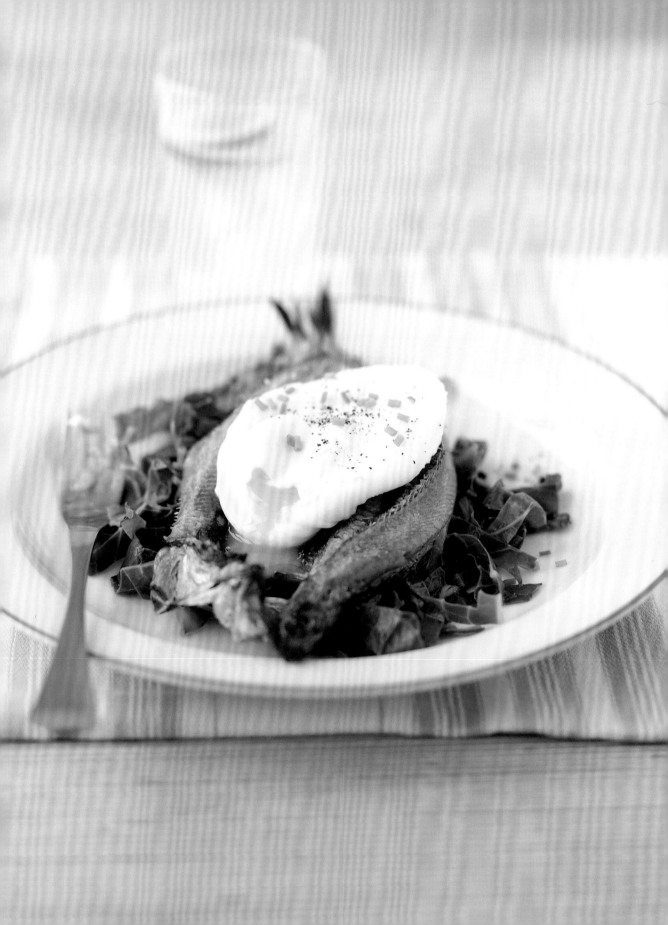

raspberry & strawberry yoghurt smoothie

This substantial fruity smoothie will keep you feeling satisfied all morning.

Ingredients

40 g (1½ oz) strawberries, hulled

40 g (1½ oz) raspberries

120 g (4 oz) low-fat Greek yoghurt

100 ml (3½ fl oz) skimmed milk

a few ice cubes

Method

1 Tip all of the ingredients into a blender or food processor and blitz until thick and creamy.

2 Serve immediately.

Tips & variations

To increase the shelf life of your fruit, portion out the berries and freeze. The fruit can be blended from frozen, which will make the smoothie thicker.

SERVINGS		NUTRITION	
0	Carbohydrates	148	Calories
0	Protein	18 g	Carbohydrates
0	Fat	11 g	Protein
1½	Dairy	4 g	Fibre
0	Vegetables	0.4 g	Salt
1	Fruit		

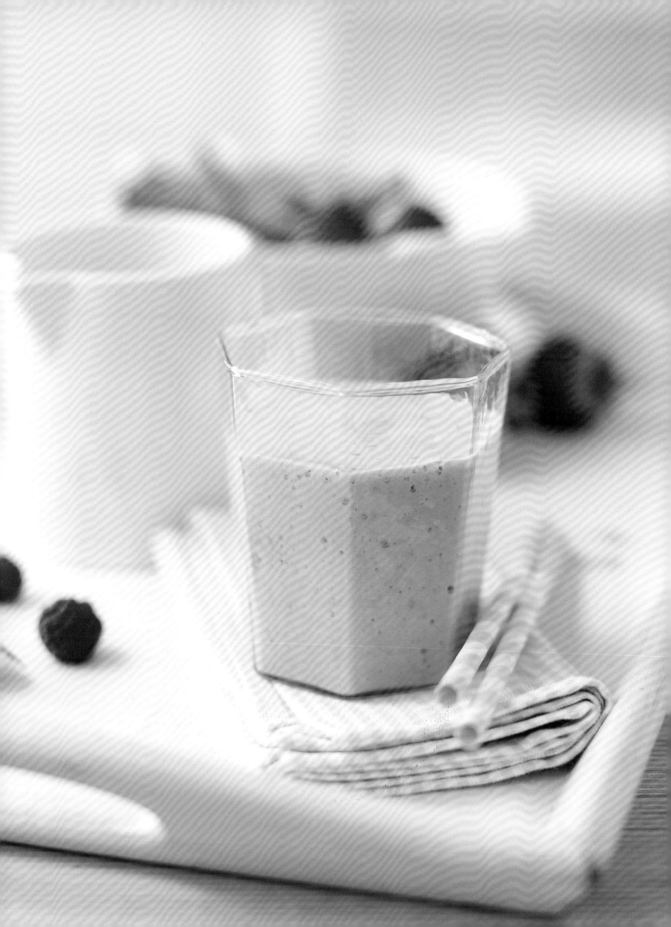

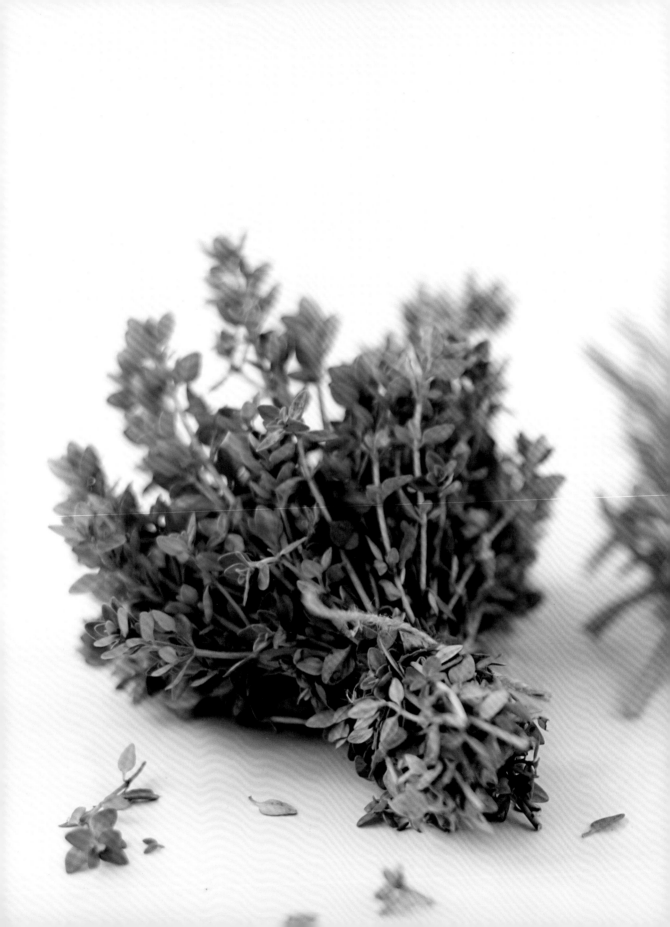

restricted days
soups

spring green soup

This delicious soup is quick to make and is bursting with fresh, spring flavours.

Ingredients

1 tsp olive oil

2 medium leeks, finely sliced

1 litre (1¾ pints) low-salt stock

180 g (6⅓ oz) frozen soya beans

160 g (5½ oz) spring greens, shredded

4 spring onions, sliced

1 tbsp thyme, leaves only

60 g (2⅓ oz) low-fat Cheddar cheese

black pepper

Method

1 Heat the oil in a large saucepan over a medium–low heat. Add the leeks and cook, stirring from time to time, until softened and golden at the edges.

2 Add the stock and bring to the boil. Add the soya beans and cook for 2 minutes.

3 Add the spring greens and cook for a further minute before ladling the soup into bowls. Scatter over the spring onions, thyme and cheese. Season with black pepper.

Tips & variations

You can freeze the soup before you add the spring onions, thyme and cheese.

SERVINGS		NUTRITION	
0	Carbohydrates	150	Calories
1½	Protein	6 g	Carbohydrates
0	Fat	14 g	Protein
½	Dairy	6 g	Fibre
1½	Vegetables	1.1 g	Salt
0	Fruit		

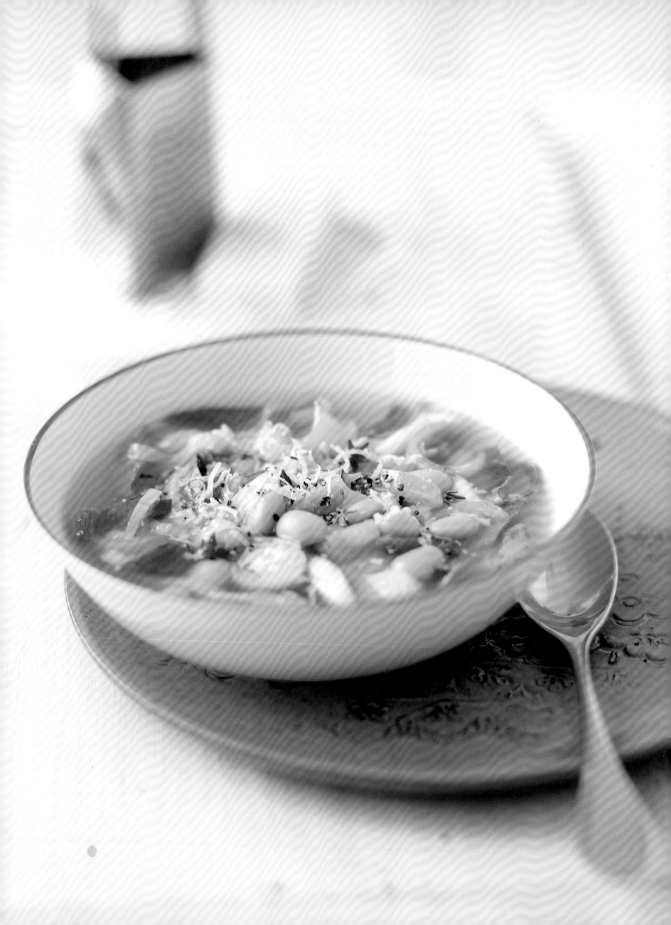

spiced pumpkin, tomato & spinach soup

This warming, gently spiced soup will give you a nice toasty feeling on cold, wintry days.

Ingredients

1 tsp olive oil

2 cloves garlic, crushed

½ tsp each ground cinnamon, cumin and coriander

chilli flakes, pinch

300 g (10½ oz) pumpkin, peeled and cut into 1-cm (½-in) dice

1 tin tomatoes, chopped

1 litre (1¾ pints) low-salt vegetable stock

150 g (5 oz) baby spinach

2 tbsp coriander, roughly chopped

black pepper

Method

1 Heat the oil in a large saucepan over a medium heat. Add the garlic, along with the spices and the chilli, and cook for 1 minute, until fragrant.

2 Add the pumpkin and cook for a further minute, until it is coated in spices and beginning to colour.

3 Pour in the tomatoes, followed by the stock and bring to the boil. Lower the heat and simmer for 15–20 minutes, until the pumpkin is tender.

4 Stir in the spinach and cook for 1 minute, until wilted, before ladling into bowls. Season to taste with black pepper and serve scattered with coriander.

Tips & variations

This soup is perfect for freezing before you add the coriander leaves. If you're not a fan of chillies, omit the chilli flakes.

SERVINGS			NUTRITION	
0	Carbohydrates		52	Calories
0	Protein		6 g	Carbohydrates
0	Fat		3 g	Protein
0	Dairy		3 g	Fibre
2	Vegetables		1.1 g	Salt
0	Fruit			

Indonesian chicken soup

Aromatic and delicious, this soup is a lighter version of Indonesian favourite, soto ayam.

Ingredients

240 g (8½ oz) chicken breast, chopped into bite-sized pieces

½ tsp each ground turmeric, coriander and cumin

2 cloves garlic, crushed

2.5-cm (1-in) piece ginger, peeled and finely grated

1 stick lemon grass, finely sliced, woody outer leaves removed

1 tsp rapeseed oil

1 litre (1¾ pints) low-salt chicken stock

2 eggs

150 g (5 oz) beansprouts

4 spring onions, finely sliced

1 lime, quartered

1 red chilli, finely sliced

2 tbsp coriander leaves, roughly chopped

black pepper

Method

1 Begin by placing the chicken in a mixing bowl and scattering over the spices, garlic, ginger and lemon grass. Grind over a good pinch of black pepper and set aside for a minimum of 1 hour, or overnight, to marinate.

2 Heat the oil in a large saucepan over a medium heat. Add the chicken, along with all of the marinade and fry, turning every so often, for 3–4 minutes, until the spices are fragrant and the chicken is nicely golden.

3 Add the stock, bring to a simmer and cook for 5–8 minutes until the chicken is cooked though.

4 Meanwhile, boil the eggs in a separate pan for 8 minutes, peel and set aside.

5 Add the beansprouts and spring onions to the soup and immediately ladle into bowls. Serve with half a boiled egg floating in each bowl, a wedge of lime on the side and the chilli and coriander divided between each bowl.

Tips & variations

You can freeze this soup at the stage when the chicken is cooked through. Boil the eggs and add the beansprouts when you reheat to serve.

SERVINGS		NUTRITION	
0	Carbohydrates	143	Calories
2½	Protein	3 g	Carbohydrates
0	Fat	19 g	Protein
0	Dairy	1 g	Fibre
½	Vegetables	1.1 g	Salt
0	Fruit		

saffron fish soup

This soup is a healthy take on an Italian classic, flavoured with saffron and rosemary.

Ingredients

1 tsp olive oil

1 small fennel bulb, finely sliced

saffron, small pinch

1 fat clove garlic, crushed

1 litre (1¾ pints) low-salt fish stock

1 bay leaf

240 g (8½ oz) cod fillet, cut into 2.5-cm (1-in) pieces

3 medium tomatoes, finely chopped

180 g (6⅓ oz) raw king prawns, thawed, if frozen

1 tbsp rosemary, finely chopped

Method

1 Heat the oil in a large saucepan over a medium heat. Add the fennel and cook, stirring occasionally, for 6–8 minutes, until softened. You may need to add a couple of tablespoons of water if the fennel begins to catch.

2 Crumble in the saffron and add the garlic and cook for 1 minute, until aromatic.

3 Pour in the stock, adding the bay leaf. Bring to the boil and lower the heat to a simmer.

4 Add the cod and simmer for 1 minute, tip in the tomatoes and prawns and cook for a further minute.

5 Discard the bay leaf. Ladle into bowls and scatter over the rosemary.

Tips & variations

You can make the soup base of fennel, saffron, garlic, stock and bay leaf ahead of time and freeze it.

SERVINGS	
0	Carbohydrates
2	Protein
0	Fat
0	Dairy
1½	Vegetables
0	Fruit

NUTRITION	
116	Calories
4 g	Carbohydrates
20 g	Protein
3 g	Fibre
1.2 g	Salt

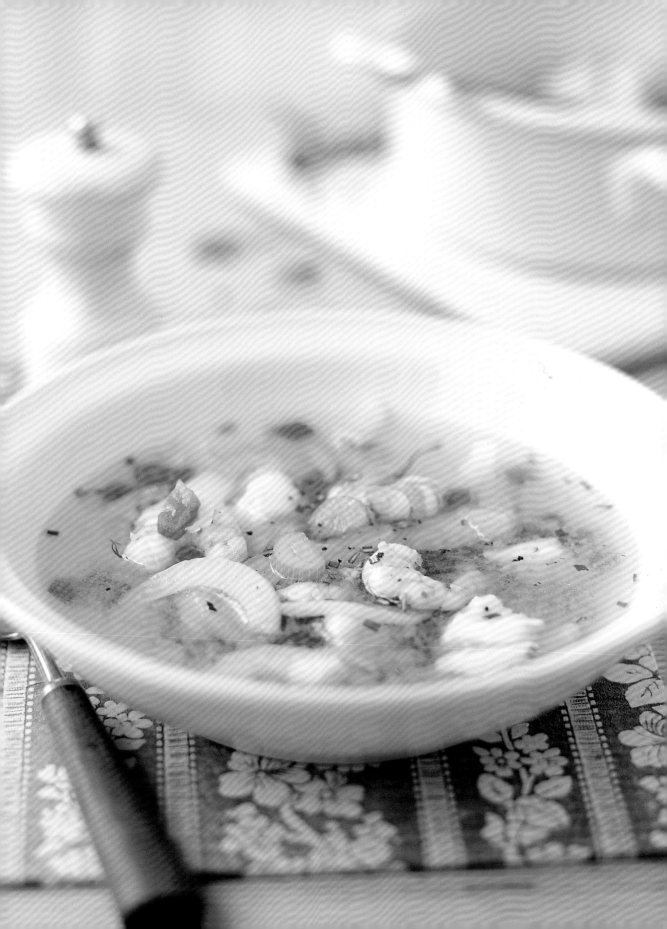

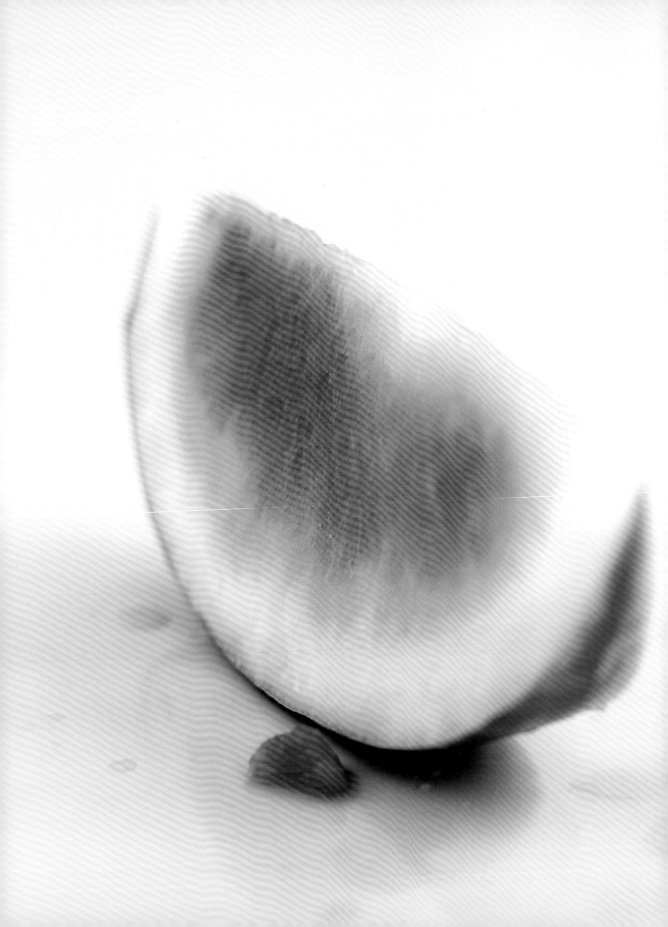

restricted days
salads & packed lunches

spring fennel salad

Refreshing, crisp and crunchy, this salad is just like springtime on a plate.

Ingredients

80 g (2½ oz) fennel bulb, finely sliced (using a mandolin if you have one), fronds reserved

½ tsp fennel seeds

1 tsp olive oil

½ lemon, juice

1 stick celery, finely sliced

5 radishes, finely sliced

60 g (2 oz) soya beans, thawed if frozen and blanched in boiling water for 3 minutes

baby salad leaves, handful

black pepper

Method

1 Tip the fennel into a bowl, scatter over the fennel seeds and sprinkle with the olive oil and lemon juice. Season with black pepper and set aside for five minutes.

2 Add the remaining ingredients, including the reserved fennel fronds and toss to coat.

Tips & variations

If you don't have a mandolin, cutting the fennel in half first will make it easier to slice.

SERVINGS		NUTRITION	
0	Carbohydrates	135	Calories
2	Protein	6 g	Carbohydrates
½	Fat	10 g	Protein
0	Dairy	8 g	Fibre
2½	Vegetables	<0.1 g	Salt
0	Fruit		

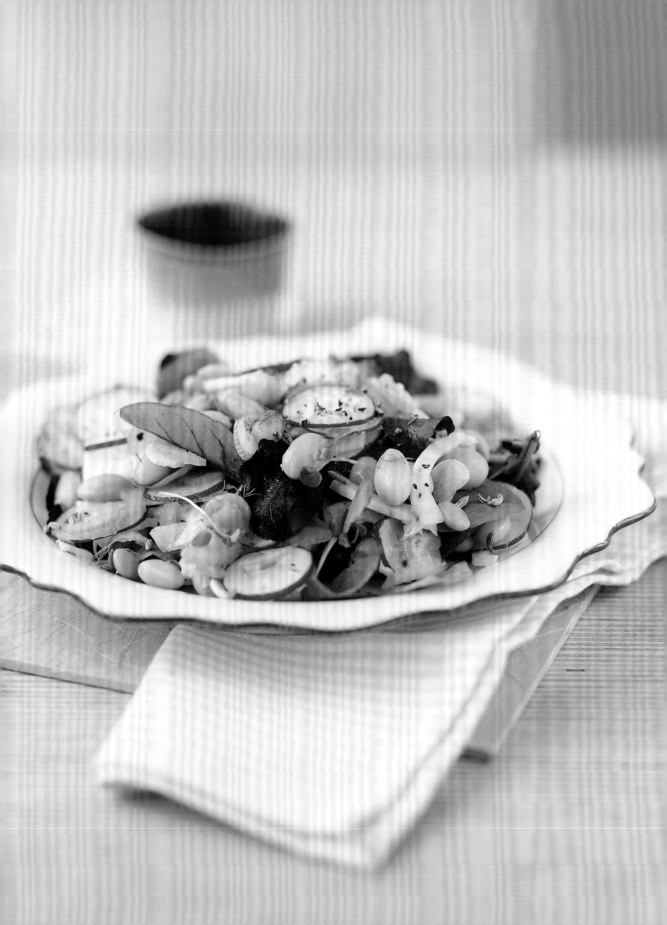

halloumi, watermelon & mint salad

A perfect marriage of fresh, sweet and savoury Greek flavours.

Ingredients

60 g (2 oz) low-fat halloumi, cut into slices

1 tsp olive oil

80 g (2¾ oz) watermelon, cut into bite-sized pieces

cos lettuce leaves, approximate handful, roughly torn

5 Kalamata olives, stoned, roughly chopped

1 tsp lemon juice

2 tsp mint leaves, roughly torn

black pepper

Method

1 Place a griddle pan or heavy non-stick frying pan over a high heat. Toss the halloumi in a bowl with the oil and when the griddle is smoking hot, add the halloumi. Cook for 1 minute before turning over with tongs.

2 Remove the halloumi from the griddle and return it to the oiled bowl.

3 Toss the halloumi with the remaining ingredients and season with black pepper.

Tips & variations

Feta makes a delicious, tangy alternative to halloumi and is just as authentically Greek. If you can't find Kalamata olives, just use any black olives.

SERVINGS		NUTRITION	
0	Carbohydrates	224	Calories
0	Protein	7 g	Carbohydrates
1	Fat	10 g	Protein
2	Dairy	2 g	Fibre
½	Vegetables	2.3 g	Salt
1	Fruit		

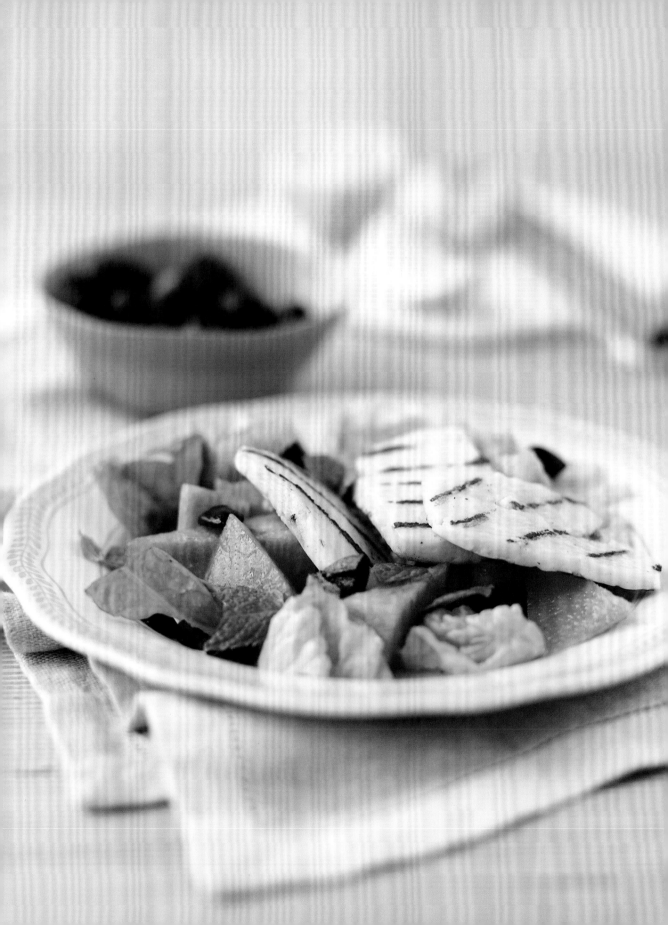

tofu & mushroom lettuce spring rolls

These fresh and tasty wraps offer a great alternative to ordinary sandwiches.

Ingredients

100 g (3½ oz) firm tofu, drained and patted dry, cut in half horizontally into 2 slabs

1-cm (½-in) piece ginger, peeled and finely grated

1 tsp low-salt soy sauce

½ lime, juice

½ tsp sesame seeds

80 g (2¾ oz) mixed mushrooms

2–4 large, soft lettuce leaves (butterhead is a good variety)

8 chives

Method

1 Place the tofu in a bowl and add the ginger, soy sauce and lime. Cover the tofu with the marinade and set aside for 30 minutes or overnight.

2 Place a non-stick frying pan over a medium heat. Remove the tofu from the marinade and scatter over the sesame seeds. Cook for 1 minute before turning over, adding the remaining marinade and mushrooms for the other minute of cooking time. Carefully remove the tofu and mushrooms from the pan and set aside to cool.

3 Lay the lettuce leaves out on a chopping board (if 1 leaf is not large enough to encase 1 piece of tofu, lay out 2 overlapping leaves for each tofu piece). Place 1 piece of tofu and half the mushrooms in the centre of each lettuce leaf, top with 4 chives each and carefully roll up to encase the filling. Secure with a cocktail stick, if necessary, and serve.

Tips & variations

You can use dried mushrooms instead of fresh – use 2 tablespoons of dried mushrooms, soak in 4 tablespoons of boiling water for 10 minutes and drain before using.

SERVINGS		NUTRITION	
0	Carbohydrates	116	Calories
2	Protein	2 g	Carbohydrates
½	Fat	11 g	Protein
0	Dairy	3 g	Fibre
1½	Vegetables	0.2 g	Salt
0	Fruit		

smoked mackerel, egg & watercress salad

with a horseradish dressing

This easy-to-prepare salad is packed full of rich flavours, so give yourself a treat.

Ingredients

1 egg

90 g (3 oz) smoked mackerel, skin removed

5 radishes, finely sliced

watercress, handful, woody stalks removed

1 tsp toasted almonds

1 tsp horseradish sauce

2 tsp lemon juice

Method

1 Place the egg in a pan of boiling water and allow to simmer for 7 minutes.

2 Carefully drain the egg and transfer it to a bowl of ice-cold water. Set aside for 10 minutes.

3 Meanwhile flake the mackerel and toss it with the radishes, watercress and almonds.

4 To serve the salad, peel the egg and cut it into quarters. Top the salad with the egg, mix the horseradish with the lemon juice and drizzle over the salad.

Tips & variations

You can use peppered smoked mackerel instead of plain if you prefer. For a vegetarian alternative you can use 60 g (2 oz) frozen soya beans (2 servings of protein) or 80 g (2¾ oz) asparagus (1 additional serving of vegetables). Blanch the soya beans for 3 minutes and allow to cool.

SERVINGS		NUTRITION	
0	Carbohydrates	471	Calories
4	Protein	3 g	Carbohydrates
½	Fat	28 g	Protein
0	Dairy	2 g	Fibre
1	Vegetables	2.3 g	Salt
0	Fruit		

crab, melon & rocket salad

This robust and refreshing salad uses lively flavours to complement the crab meat.

Ingredients

90 g (3 oz) white crab meat

1-cm (½-in) piece root ginger, peeled and finely grated

2 tsp lime juice

½ red chilli, de-seeded and finely chopped

1 tsp rapeseed oil

80 g (2¾ oz) cantaloupe or other orange-fleshed melon, cut into bite-sized pieces

rocket leaves, handful

1 tsp each mint and coriander, roughly torn

Method

1 Spoon the crab meat into a bowl and scatter over the ginger, lime juice and chilli – toss to coat.

2 Add the remaining ingredients and lightly toss until completely coated in dressing. Serve cold.

Tips & variations

Fresh white crab meat is available at most supermarkets. You can also use tinned crab meat. For a vegetarian option replace the crab meat with 30 g (1 oz) feta cheese (0 servings of protein, 1 serving of dairy).

SERVINGS		NUTRITION	
0	Carbohydrates	173	Calories
2	Protein	5 g	Carbohydrates
½	Fat	20 g	Protein
0	Dairy	2 g	Fibre
½	Vegetables	1.1 g	Salt
1	Fruit		

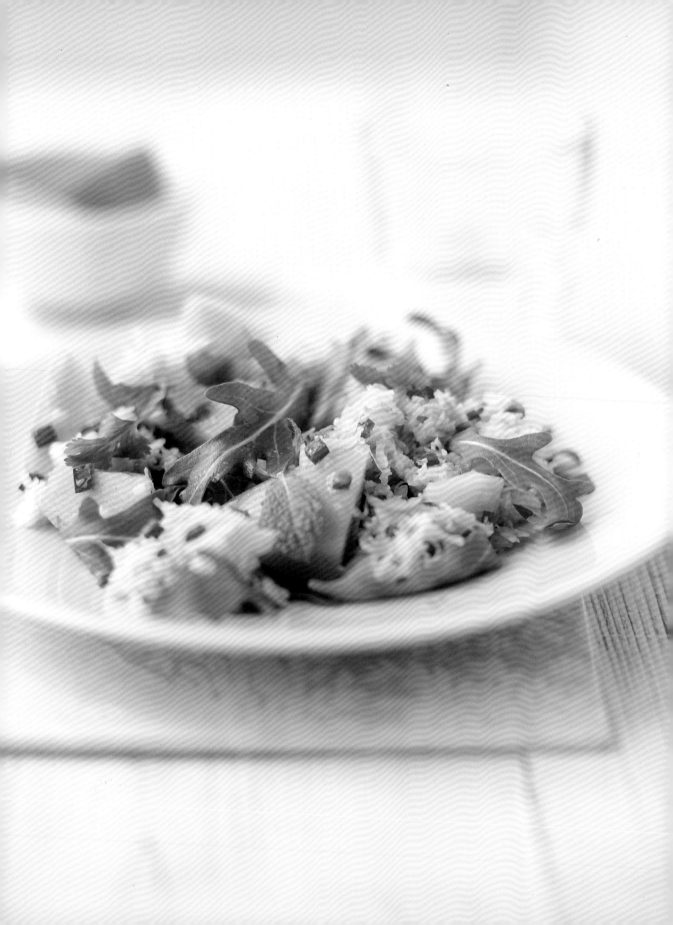

bang bang chicken salad

This fiery salad is based on the classic szechuan dish with a tangy peanut dressing.

Ingredients

500 ml (17½ fl oz) low-salt chicken stock

120 g (4 oz) skinless chicken breast

1 tsp peanut butter

½ tsp low-salt soy sauce

¼ tsp fish sauce

½ tsp rice vinegar

1-cm (½-in) piece ginger, peeled and
    finely grated

½ red chilli, de-seeded and finely chopped

80 g (2¾ oz) Chinese leaves, shredded

5-cm (2-in) piece cucumber, finely sliced

5 radishes, finely sliced

2 spring onions, finely sliced

1 tsp each mint and coriander, roughly
    chopped

Method

1 Begin by bringing the stock to the boil in a small saucepan over a medium heat. Add the chicken breast, lower the heat to a simmer and poach the chicken for 10–15 minutes, until cooked through. Remove from the pan and set aside to cool. Reserve 1 tablespoon of the stock when you remove the chicken.

2 When the chicken is cool enough to handle, shred into bite-sized pieces.

3 Toss the chicken with the peanut butter, soy sauce, fish sauce, vinegar, ginger and chilli until coated in the dressing. Add the tablespoon of reserved stock to loosen.

4 Serve the chicken on a bed of the Chinese leaves, cucumber and radishes and scatter the spring onions and herbs over the top.

Tips & variations

The dressing freezes well and also goes beautifully with pork and beef. For a vegetarian alternative use 115 g (4 oz) Quorn pieces (4 servings of protein), low-salt vegetable stock and increase the soy sauce to replace the fish sauce. Heat the Quorn through for 5 minutes in the stock before continuing to step 2. If you don't have rice vinegar you can use white wine vinegar instead.

SERVINGS		NUTRITION	
0	Carbohydrates	219	Calories
4	Protein	6 g	Carbohydrates
1	Fat	31 g	Protein
0	Dairy	3 g	Fibre
2½	Vegetables	2 g	Salt
0	Fruit		

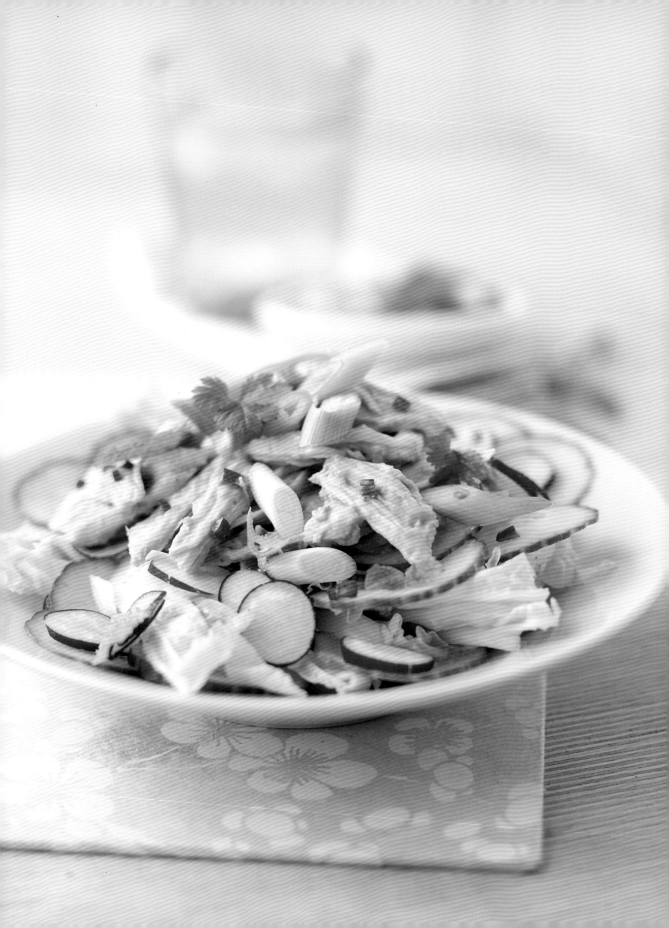

green bean, broccoli & chicken salad

A light and versatile salad – the perfect choice for a summer picnic.

Ingredients

½ lemon, juice and zest

1 tsp olive oil

1 clove garlic, crushed

120 g (4 oz) skinless chicken breast

1 tsp mixed seeds

80 g (2¾ oz) tenderstem broccoli, woody ends trimmed

80 g (2¾ oz) fine green beans, trimmed

1 little gem lettuce, shredded

1 tsp flat-leaf parsley, roughly chopped

black pepper

Method

1 Preheat the oven to 200°C/400°F/gas mark 6. Rub half of the lemon juice and zest, half the oil and the garlic over the chicken breast.

2 Season with black pepper and place on a roasting tin. Roast for 15–20 minutes, scattering over the seeds for the last 3 minutes of cooking, until the chicken is golden brown and the juices run clear. Set aside to cool.

3 Meanwhile, blanch the broccoli and the beans in boiling water for 2 minutes. Then drain and run under cold water to refresh. Toss with the lettuce, the remaining lemon juice and zest.

4 When the chicken has cooled, shred into bite-sized pieces and toss with the salad. Scatter over the parsley.

Tips & variations

When in season, purple sprouting broccoli makes a great alternative to the tenderstem kind.

SERVINGS			NUTRITION	
0	Carbohydrates		245	Calories
4	Protein		7 g	Carbohydrates
1	Fat		34 g	Protein
0	Dairy		7 g	Fibre
3	Vegetables		0.3 g	Salt
0	Fruit			

pesto turkey salad

This salad uses classic Italian flavours to liven up the simplicity of turkey.

Ingredients

120 g (4 oz) turkey breast, chopped into 1-cm (½-in) pieces

¼ tsp olive oil

1 small clove garlic, crushed

1 tsp green pesto

160 g (5½ oz) cherry tomatoes, halved

salad leaves, handful

basil leaves, small handful, roughly torn

1 tsp balsamic vinegar

black pepper

Method

1 Preheat the oven to 200°C/400°F/gas mark 6. Toss the turkey with the oil and garlic. Season with pepper and transfer to a small ovenproof dish.

2 Roast in the oven for 8–10 minutes, until the pieces are cooked through.

3 Remove from the oven and toss with the remaining ingredients. Serve warm, or if serving cold, wait until the chicken has cooled before combining with the salad leaves, basil and balsamic vinegar.

Tips & variations

Fresh green pesto is available in most large supermarkets. Look out for rocket pesto as a fiery alternative to the usual kind. Use normal pesto in a jar if fresh pesto is not available.

SERVINGS		NUTRITION	
0	Carbohydrates	209	Calories
4	Protein	7 g	Carbohydrates
1	Fat	32 g	Protein
0	Dairy	3 g	Fibre
2½	Vegetables	0.5 g	Salt
0	Fruit		

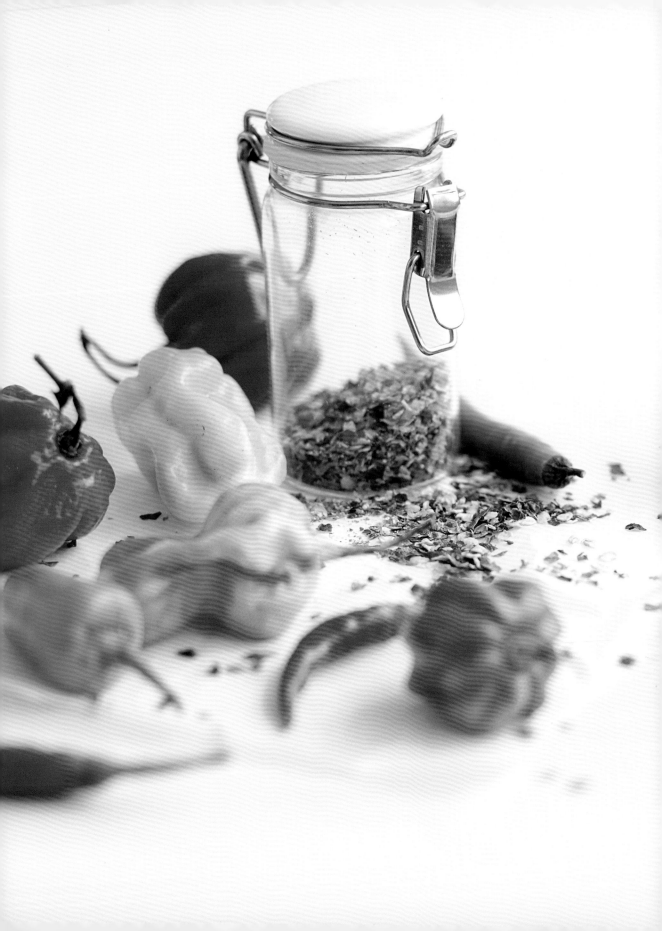

restricted days
30-minute meals

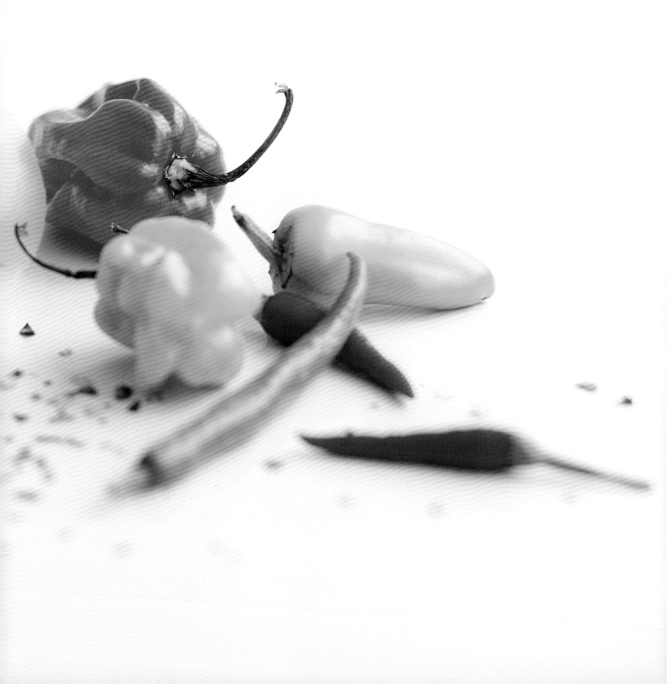

piri piri turkey & green pepper skewers with a tomato salad

These Portuguese-spiced skewers are a great alternative to ordinary piri piri chicken.

Ingredients

FOR THE SKEWERS

240 g (8½ oz) turkey breast, cut into
   2.5-cm (1-in) pieces

2 green peppers, de-seeded and cut into
   2.5-cm (1-in) chunks

2 cloves garlic, crushed

2 tsp smoked paprika

1 lemon, juice

2 tsp Worcester sauce

1 tsp thyme, leaves only, roughly chopped

black pepper

FOR THE SALAD

320 g (11 oz) cherry tomatoes, halved

½ lemon, juice

160 g (5½ oz) rocket leaves

basil leaves, bunch

Method

1. Preheat the grill to high. Soak 8 wooden skewers in hot water and set aside for 10 minutes.

2. Place the turkey and peppers in a bowl and scatter over the garlic, paprika, lemon juice, Worcester sauce and thyme leaves. Season with pepper and stir everything until completely covered in sauce.

3. Divide the turkey and peppers between the skewers, carefully sliding them on. Once complete, transfer them to a grill pan. Grill for 10–12 minutes, turning halfway through the cooking time, until the turkey is cooked through.

4. Meanwhile combine the salad ingredients and transfer to a salad bowl for serving.

5. Serve 2 skewers per person, accompanied by a generous helping of tomato salad and a sprinkling of black pepper.

Tips & variations

You can marinate the turkey in the piri piri sauce a day ahead to give it a really intense flavour. For a vegetarian alternative marinate 230 g (8 oz) Quorn fillets cut into large chunks (2 servings of protein) and use vegetarian Worcester sauce or soy sauce.

SERVINGS		NUTRITION	
0	Carbohydrates	107	Calories
2	Protein	7 g	Carbohydrates
0	Fat	18 g	Protein
0	Dairy	3 g	Fibre
2½	Vegetables	0.3 g	Salt
0	Fruit		

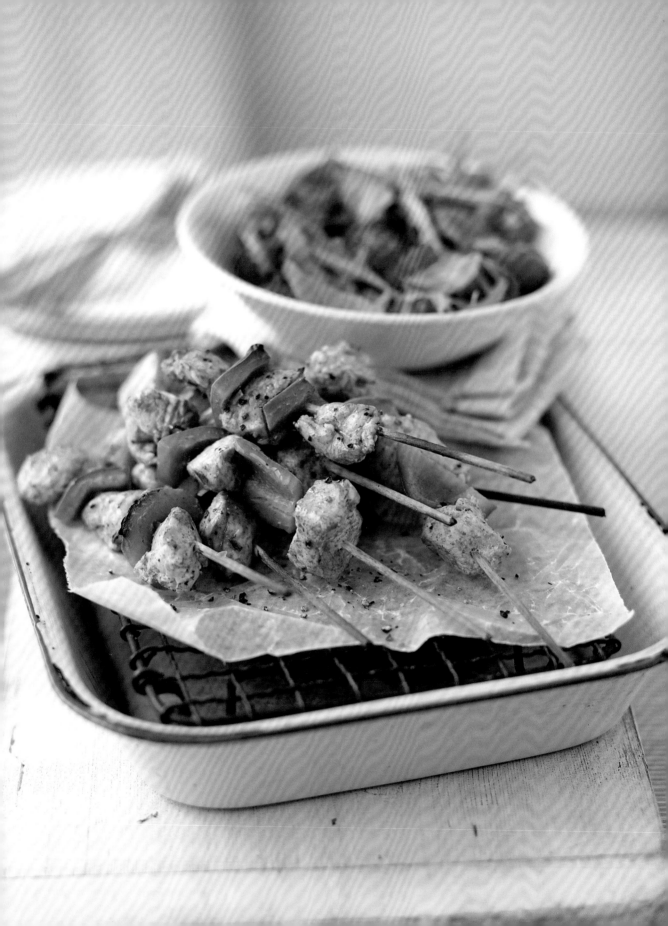

open spiced turkey burgers

with guacamole topping

The piquant spices in these burgers are cut through by the creamy but sharp guacamole.

Ingredients

FOR THE BURGERS

480 g (1 lb 1 oz) turkey mince

2 tsp harissa paste

4 spring onions, finely sliced

1 tbsp coriander, roughly chopped

1 tbsp mint, roughly chopped

1 egg yolk

2 tsp olive oil

black pepper

FOR THE GUACAMOLE

1 avocado

1 medium tomato, roughly diced

2 spring onions, finely sliced

½ lime, juice

2 Little Gem lettuces, leaves

coriander leaves, small handful

Method

1 Begin by making the burger patties. In a large bowl mix together the turkey mince, harissa paste, spring onions, coriander, mint and egg yolk. Season with black pepper and continue to mix until all of the ingredients are combined.

2 Divide the mixture into 8 and form into equal-sized patties. Place on a plate lined with baking parchment and refrigerate for 30 minutes.

3 Preheat the oven to 200°C/400°F/gas mark 6, remove the patties from the fridge and heat the oil in a large frying pan over a medium heat. Once the oil is hot, fry the patties in batches for 2–3 minutes on each side, until nicely golden. Transfer to a baking tray and cook for 10–15 minutes, until cooked through.

4 To make the guacamole topping, cut the avocado in half and remove the stone. Scoop out the flesh and cut into long slices. Carefully combine with the tomato, spring onions and lime juice. To assemble the burgers, lay 2 patties per person on a bed of lettuce leaves. Top with guacamole and scatter over the coriander.

Tips & variations

To save time, make and shape the patties the day before you want to eat them and store them in the fridge. This will also help the burgers maintain their shape.

SERVINGS		NUTRITION	
0	Carbohydrates	255	Calories
4	Protein	2 g	Carbohydrates
1	Fat	32 g	Protein
0	Dairy	3 g	Fibre
½	Vegetables	1 g	Salt
0	Fruit		

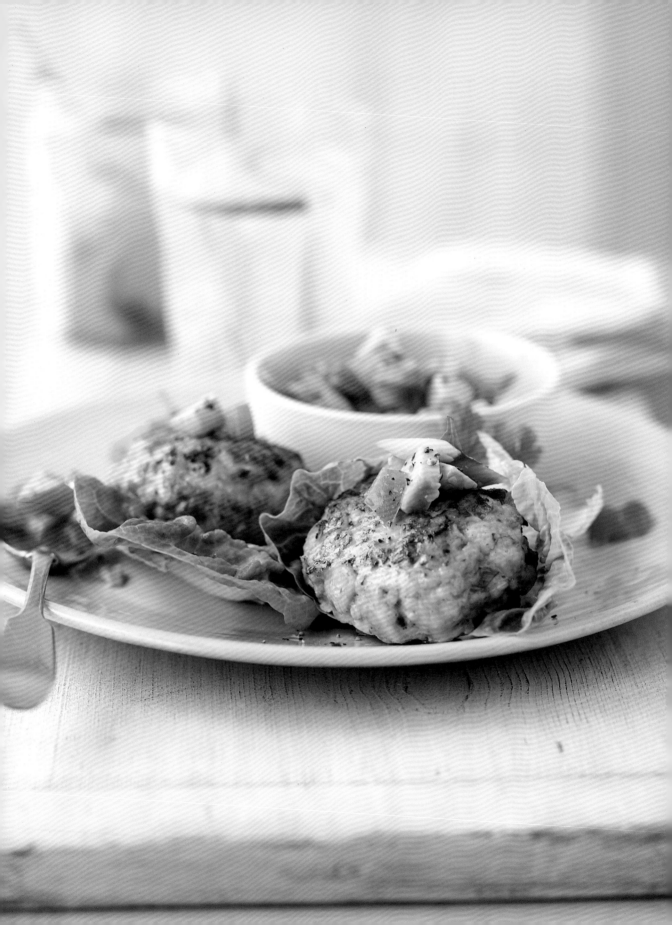

grilled miso chicken

with pickled vegetable salad

This Japanese-inspired recipe combines richly savoury miso with sharp, pickled vegetables.

Ingredients

4 skinless chicken breasts, approximately 120 g (4 oz) each

1 tbsp miso paste

1 tbsp low-salt soy sauce

2.5-cm (1-in) piece root ginger, peeled and finely grated

3 tbsp rice or white wine vinegar

½ lime, juice

chilli flakes, pinch

1 tsp sesame oil

160 g (5½ oz) Chinese leaves, shredded

20 radishes, finely sliced

10-cm (4-in) piece cucumber, cut into sticks

160 g (5½ oz) mangetout, sliced in half

1 tsp sesame seeds, toasted

2 tbsp coriander leaves

Method

1 Place the chicken breasts on a board and using a sharp knife, make 3–4 diagonal slashes about 1 cm (½ in) deep on each piece of chicken.

2 Transfer to a bowl and cover with the miso paste, soy sauce, ginger and 1 tablespoon of the vinegar. Set aside for 10 minutes.

3 Meanwhile, preheat the grill to medium. To prepare the pickled vegetable salad, combine the remaining ingredients (apart from the coriander) in a bowl and set aside to marinate.

4 Place the chicken breasts in a grill pan and grill for 15–20 minutes, turning halfway through, until completely cooked through.

5 To serve, slice the chicken into 1-cm (½-in) slices and serve on a bed of the pickled vegetable salad. Scatter with the coriander leaves.

Tips & variations

You can store the pickled vegetable salad, covered, in the fridge for 2 days before serving. For a vegetarian alternative use 1 packet of firm tofu (approximately 400 g/14 oz), sliced into 4, marinated in the sauce and grilled or fried until crisp around the edges.

SERVINGS		NUTRITION	
0	Carbohydrates	189	Calories
4	Protein	5 g	Carbohydrates
0	Fat	30 g	Protein
0	Dairy	3 g	Fibre
2	Vegetables	0.9 g	Salt
0	Fruit		

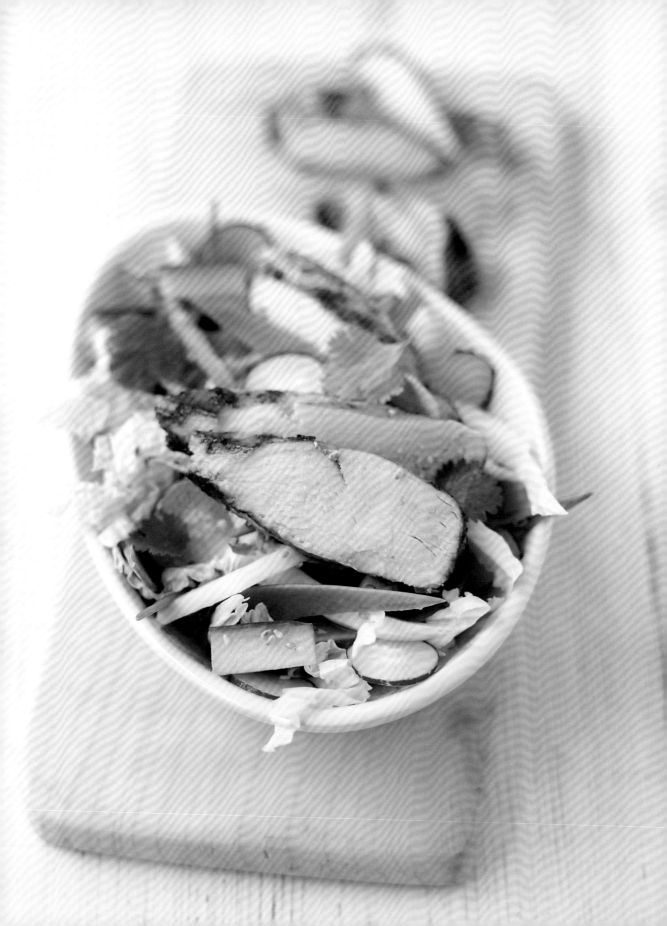

stuffed tarragon chicken

with bacon & roasted vegetables

Chicken and tarragon make a classic combination for a restricted day.

Ingredients

4 skinless chicken breasts, approximately 120 g (4 oz) each

4 tbsp low-fat cream cheese

2 cloves garlic, crushed

1 tbsp tarragon, roughly chopped

4 rashers lean bacon

160 g (5½ oz) asparagus spears, woody ends trimmed

160 g (5½ oz) courgette, cut into 1-cm (½-in) slices

2 tsp olive oil

½ lemon, juice

chilli flakes, pinch

black pepper

Method

1 Preheat the oven to 200°C/400°F/gas mark 6. Place the chicken breasts on a board and carefully cut a 2.5-cm (1-in) pocket into the side of each piece.

2 Beat together the cream cheese, garlic and tarragon, season with pepper and carefully spoon a quarter of the stuffing mixture into each chicken breast. Pinch the seams of the cut flesh together and carefully wrap each breast in a piece of bacon.

3 Place the chicken breast, seam-side down, on a baking tray and roast for 20 minutes, until cooked through.

4 Toss the vegetables in the oil, lemon juice and chilli flakes and roast in the oven for the final 10–12 minutes of cooking time, until golden brown.

Tips & variations

You can stuff the chicken, wrap it in the bacon and then freeze it ahead of time. You can also serve with additional steamed vegetables on the side.

SERVINGS		NUTRITION	
0	Carbohydrates	278	Calories
5	Protein	3 g	Carbohydrates
0	Fat	39 g	Protein
1	Dairy	1 g	Fibre
1	Vegetables	1.7 g	Salt
0	Fruit		

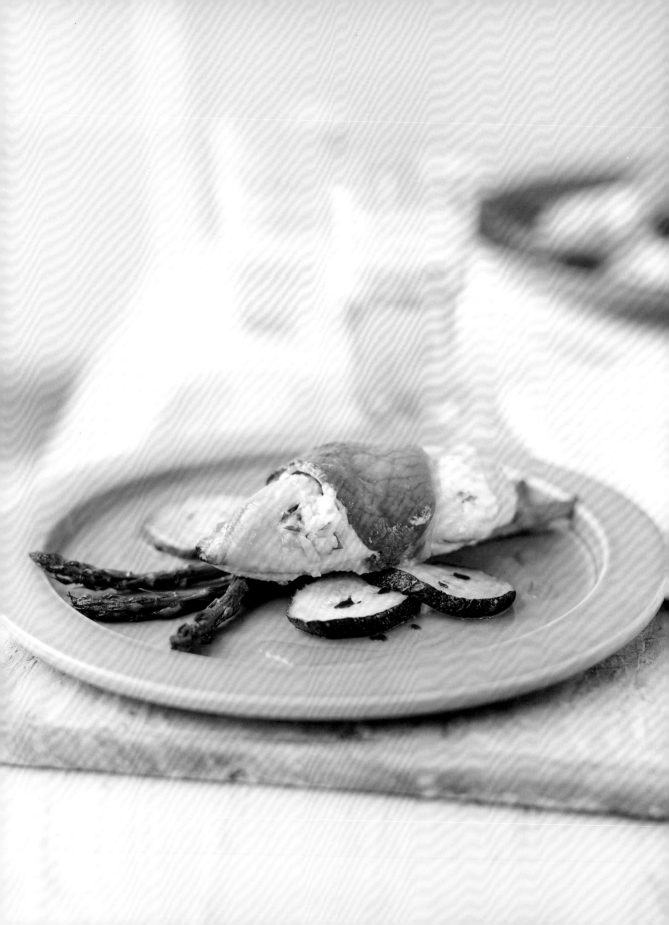

chicken & spinach curry

with raita

This spicy dish is as satisfying as a traditional curry, but it's light on calories.

Ingredients

FOR THE CURRY

1 tsp olive oil

480 g (1 lb 1 oz) chicken breast, cut into 2.5-cm (1-in) pieces

2.5-cm (1-in) piece ginger, peeled and finely grated

2 cloves garlic, crushed

2 tsp ground coriander

2 tsp ground cumin

1 tsp ground turmeric

1 tsp chilli powder

1 tin chopped tomatoes

100 ml (3½ fl oz) low-salt chicken stock

160 g (5½ oz) medium okra

160 g (5²/₃ oz) baby spinach

coriander leaves, handful

1 lemon, cut into wedges

FOR THE RAITA

300 g (10½ oz) low-fat Greek yoghurt

5-cm (2-in) piece cucumber

2 tbsp mint leaves, roughly torn

SERVINGS		NUTRITION	
0	Carbohydrates	242	Calories
4	Protein	12 g	Carbohydrates
0	Fat	35 g	Protein
½	Dairy	4 g	Fibre
1½	Vegetables	0.6 g	Salt
0	Fruit		

Method

1 Heat the oil in a large frying pan over a medium heat. When the oil is hot, add the chicken pieces and fry for 3–4 minutes, turning from time to time, until browned.

2 Add the ginger, garlic and spices and cook, stirring, for a minute, until fragrant.

3 Add the tomatoes and stock and bring up to a simmer. Simmer for 5 minutes, until slightly reduced.

4 Add the okra and cook for a further 2–3 minutes and check that the chicken is cooked before removing from the heat. Stir in the spinach.

5 Meanwhile slice the cucumber in half, scoop out the seeds and slice finely. Stir into the remaining raita ingredients and serve alongside the curry. Sprinkle over the coriander leaves and arrange a wedge of lemon alongside.

Tips & variations

This dish is delicious hot, but you can also serve it cold. For a vegetarian alternative use 500 g (1 lb 1 oz) extra-firm tofu cut into pieces and low-salt vegetable stock.

Asian duck, grapefruit & watercress salad

Infused with soy, star anise and grapefruit, this speedy salad makes a luxurious meal.

Ingredients

2 skinless duck breasts, approximately 240 g (8½ oz) each

2 tbsp low-salt soy sauce

2.5-cm (1-in) piece root ginger, peeled and finely grated

1 star anise (optional)

2 grapefruits

2 tsp sesame oil

4 spring onions, finely sliced

1 red chilli, de-seeded and finely sliced

10-cm (4-in) piece cucumber, cut into spears

160 g (5½ oz) watercress, woody stalks removed

2 tbsp coriander leaves

Method

1 Lay the duck breasts in a bowl and cover with the soy sauce, ginger, star anise, the juice of 1 of the grapefruits and the sesame oil. Set aside in the fridge to marinate for a minimum of 10 minutes – or overnight.

2 Preheat the grill to high. Remove the duck breasts from the marinade and transfer to a grill pan. Grill for 3 minutes on each side for medium, or up to 5 minutes each side for well done. Remove from the grill pan and set aside to rest for 10 minutes.

3 Meanwhile, pour the marinade into a saucepan and place over a medium heat. Bring to the boil and allow it to reduce for 5 minutes. Set aside to cool.

4 Carefully cut the skin from the remaining grapefruit and cut between the membranes to segment the grapefruit. Set aside.

5 Slice the duck breast into 1-cm (½-in) slices and toss with the marinade, grapefruit, spring onions, chilli, cucumber, watercress and coriander. Divide evenly into 4 and serve.

SERVINGS		NUTRITION	
0	Carbohydrates	229	Calories
4	Protein	8 g	Carbohydrates
0	Fat	27 g	Protein
0	Dairy	2.5 g	Fibre
1	Vegetables	0.7 g	Salt
1	Fruit		

griddled tuna steak

with pineapple salsa

Delicately flavoured tuna steaks are enlivened with a piquant pineapple salsa.

Ingredients

4 tuna steaks, approximately 120 g
 (4 oz) each

2 tsp olive oil

1 lime, juice

320 g (11 oz) fresh pineapple flesh,
 chopped into 1-cm (½-in) dice

1 red chilli, de-seeded, finely chopped

4 spring onions, sliced

2 tbsp coriander leaves, roughly chopped

320 g (11 oz) fine green beans, trimmed

240 g (8½ oz) salad leaves

black pepper

Method

1 Preheat a griddle pan or heavy frying pan over a medium heat. Once hot, rub the tuna steaks with the olive oil and half the lime juice and season with black pepper. Transfer the tuna steaks to the griddle pan and cook for 1 minute on each side for rare, 2 minutes on each side for medium.

2 Meanwhile, mix the remaining lime juice with the pineapple, chilli, spring onions and coriander leaves to make the salsa. Set aside.

3 Blanch the green beans in boiling water for 2 minutes. Serve the tuna steaks topped with salsa, with the beans and salad on the side.

Tips & variations

Try out some alternative flavourings: you could experiment with pesto, lime and coriander dressing or a tomato salad.

SERVINGS		NUTRITION	
0	Carbohydrates	255	Calories
4	Protein	12 g	Carbohydrates
0	Fat	31 g	Protein
0	Dairy	5 g	Fibre
2	Vegetables	0.2 g	Salt
1	Fruit		

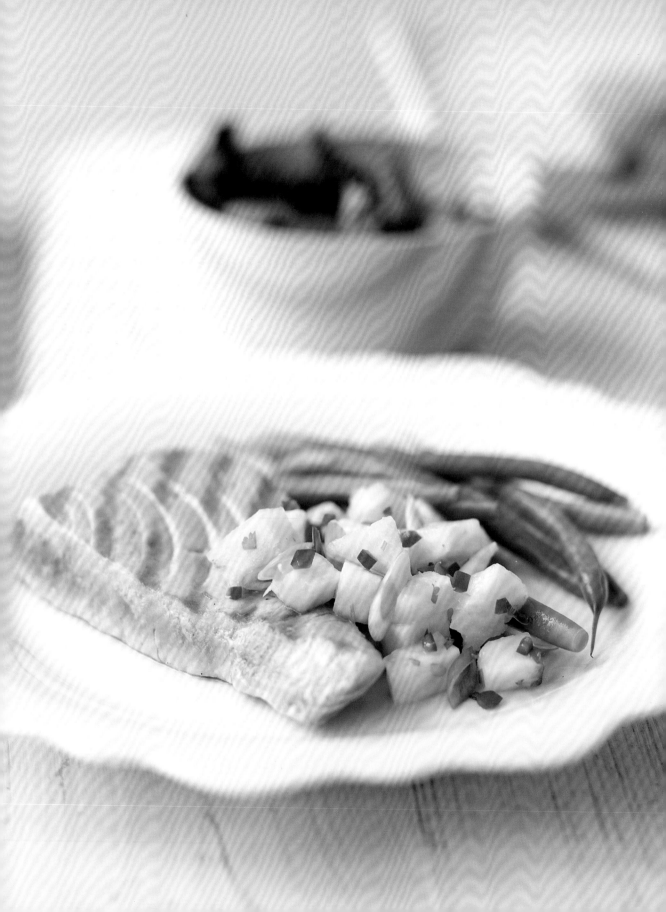

lemon & garlic tiger prawns

with crushed soya beans

Perfect for a light summer meal, these sweet and flavoursome prawns are delicious.

Ingredients

360 g (12½ oz) raw tiger prawns, thawed if frozen

1 lemon, juice and zest

2 cloves garlic, crushed

1 tbsp flat-leaf parsley, roughly chopped

240 g (8½ oz) soya beans, thawed if frozen

3 tsp olive oil

4 tsp mint leaves, roughly torn

200 g (7 oz) rocket leaves

black pepper

Method

1 Stir together the prawns, half the lemon juice and zest, the garlic and parsley. Season with black pepper, to taste, and set aside to marinate for 30 minutes.

2 Blanch the soya beans in boiling water for 2–3 minutes, until slightly softened. Drain well and mix with 2 teaspoons of the oil and the remaining lemon juice and zest. Using a fork or potato masher, mash the beans until they are almost all crushed but still have texture. Keep warm.

3 Place a large frying pan over a medium heat and when hot, add the remaining oil. Fry the prawns for 2 minutes, or until the flesh turns pink and opaque. Stir the mint into the beans, season with black pepper and serve the prawns on a bed of crushed beans and rocket.

Tips & variations

Be sure to use raw prawns because the salt levels are much lower than in the pre-cooked type. Add chilli for an extra kick and use scallops instead of prawns if you wish. Serve with salad or steamed vegetables.

SERVINGS		NUTRITION	
0	Carbohydrates	197	Calories
4	Protein	5 g	Carbohydrates
½	Fat	26 g	Protein
0	Dairy	5 g	Fibre
½	Vegetables	0.6 g	Salt
0	Fruit		

herb-stuffed trout with baked fennel

Delicately earthy trout is enlivened with plenty of fresh herbs and sweet, zesty flavours.

Ingredients

4 skinless trout fillets, approximately
   120 g (4 oz) each

160 g (5½ oz) salad leaves

FOR THE TROUT FILLING

320 g (11 oz) fennel, finely sliced

3 tsp olive oil

2 cloves garlic, crushed

1 lemon, juice and zest

2 tbsp dill leaves, roughly chopped

2 tbsp flat-leaf parsley, roughly chopped

2 tbsp tarragon, roughly chopped

1 tbsp mint, roughly chopped

6 dried apricots, finely chopped

½ tsp crushed sumac or the zest of
   1 lemon, finely grated

black pepper

Method

1 Preheat the oven to 200°C/400°F/gas mark 6. Toss the fennel with 2 teaspoons of the oil, 1 clove of garlic and half the lemon juice and zest until completely coated. Transfer to a non-stick baking tray and cook for 5 minutes.

2 Meanwhile, place the trout fillets on a board, skinned side uppermost. Mix together the herbs, the remaining garlic and oil, apricots, sumac and remaining lemon juice and zest. Season with pepper. Using a palette knife, spread the herb filling evenly over the length of each fillet.

3 To roll up the fillets, start at the thinnest ends and carefully roll towards the thick ends. Secure with cocktail sticks and place on top of the partially cooked fennel. Return to the oven and cook for 20 minutes, until the fish flakes easily when pressed lightly. Serve with the salad leaves.

Tips and variations

Sumac is a reddish-purple spice often used in Middle Eastern dishes to give a lemony flavour. If you can't find it, use lemon zest instead.

SERVINGS		NUTRITION	
0	Carbohydrates	210	Calories
4	Protein	8 g	Carbohydrates
0	Fat	26 g	Protein
0	Dairy	4 g	Fibre
1½	Vegetables	2 g	Salt
½	Fruit		

mustard salmon

with roasted leeks, asparagus & tomatoes

This French bistro-style dish is unbelievably simple to prepare — ideal for busy weekdays.

Ingredients

4 skinless salmon fillets, approximately 120 g (4 oz) each

1 tbsp wholegrain mustard

2 medium leeks, finely sliced

320 g (11oz) asparagus spears, woody ends trimmed

160 g (5½ oz) cherry tomatoes

2 tsp olive oil

1 lemon, ½ juice and ½ wedges

1 tbsp flat-leaf parsley, roughly chopped

black pepper

Method

1 Preheat the oven to 200°C/400°F/gas mark 6. Place the salmon fillets on a board and spread with an even amount of mustard. Season with a little black pepper and transfer to a non-stick baking tray.

2 Toss the leeks, asparagus and tomatoes in the oil. Squeeze the juice of half the lemon over the vegetables and combine. Cut the remaining lemon half into 4 wedges.

3 Tuck the vegetables around the salmon fillets and bake in the oven for 20–25 minutes, until the salmon is cooked through and the vegetables are golden brown. Serve sprinkled with the parsley and with lemon wedges on the side.

Tips & variations

You can rub the salmon with the mustard and then refrigerate it overnight or freeze it.

SERVINGS		NUTRITION	
0	Carbohydrates	290	Calories
4	Protein	6 g	Carbohydrates
0	Fat	29 g	Protein
0	Dairy	5 g	Fibre
2½	Vegetables	0.5 g	Salt
0	Fruit		

baked smoked haddock

with poached egg & spiced spinach

This lighter take on kedgeree retains all the comforting flavours while bypassing the carbs.

Ingredients

4 undyed, skinless, boneless smoked haddock fillets about 150 g (5 oz) each

4 black peppercorns

2 bay leaves

1 stick celery, roughly chopped

4 eggs

2 tsp olive oil

2.5 cm (1 in) ginger, peeled and finely grated

1 clove garlic, crushed

1 tsp curry powder

4 curry leaves, dried or fresh

320 g (11 oz) baby leaf spinach, washed

2 tbsp flat-leaf parsley, roughly chopped

1 lemon, in wedges

Tips & variations

For a vegetarian alternative use 150 g (5 oz) fried, smoked tofu (3 servings of protein).

SERVINGS		NUTRITION	
0	Carbohydrates	252	Calories
3½	Protein	2 g	Carbohydrates
0	Fat	39 g	Protein
0	Dairy	2 g	Fibre
1	Vegetables	3.4 g	Salt
0	Fruit		

Method

1 Preheat the oven to 200°C/400°F/gas mark 6. Place the haddock fillets in an ovenproof dish and pour over enough freshly boiled water to just cover them. Drop the peppercorns, bay leaves and celery into the water and transfer to the oven. Bake for 15–20 minutes, until the fish flakes easily when pressed lightly. Remove the fillets from the dish and keep warm. Discard the aromatics.

2 While the fish is cooking, poach the eggs. Bring a pan of water to the boil and create a whirlpool by stirring with a wooden spoon and crack an egg into the middle of it. Turn the heat down and simmer for 4 minutes. Drain well and keep on one side. Repeat with the other eggs.

3 For the spiced spinach, heat the oil in a large frying pan over a medium heat. Add the ginger, garlic and curry powder and cook, stirring, for 1 minute, until fragrant. Crumble in the curry leaves and cook for a further minute. Pour in a couple of tablespoons of water and add the spinach. It may seem like a lot of spinach, but it will wilt down quickly. Toss the spinach in the spices for 1–2 minutes, until it is just wilted.

4 To serve, lay each haddock fillet on a bed of spinach and top with a poached egg. Sprinkle with parsley and serve with lemon wedges.

Goan spiced mackerel

with tomato & chilli sambal & raita

Rich, oily mackerel is robust enough to handle a little heat and spice. The cucumber yoghurt cools and refreshes.

Ingredients

FOR THE MACKEREL

4 fresh mackerel fillets, about 120 g (4 oz) each

½ tsp ground cumin

½ tsp ground coriander

½ tsp ground turmeric

½ tsp ground cinnamon

1 lime, juice and zest

160 g (5½ oz) salad leaves, to serve

FOR THE SAMBAL

2 red chillies

1 clove garlic

2 medium tomatoes, roughly chopped

FOR THE RAITA

300 g (10½ oz) low-fat Greek yoghurt

10-cm (4-in) piece cucumber, finely chopped

2 tbsp mint leaves, roughly chopped

Method

1 Preheat the grill to high. Rub the mackerel fillets with the spices and sprinkle with half the lime juice and zest. Grill the fillets for 4 minutes on each side, until cooked through.

2 Meanwhile, make the sambal by pounding the red chillies and garlic with a pestle and mortar. Stir in the remaining lime juice and zest, along with the tomatoes.

3 To make the raita, combine the ingredients and set aside.

4 Serve the mackerel fillets topped with the sambal. Serve the raita and salad leaves on the side.

Tips & variations

The sambal is extremely versatile and would make a wonderful accompaniment to any grilled meat, fish or even tofu. You can substitute the Greek yoghurt in the raita for plain yoghurt or low-fat fromage frais if you prefer.

SERVINGS		NUTRITION	
0	Carbohydrates	347	Calories
4	Protein	9 g	Carbohydrates
0	Fat	28 g	Protein
½	Dairy	2 g	Fibre
1½	Vegetables	0.4 g	Salt
0	Fruit		

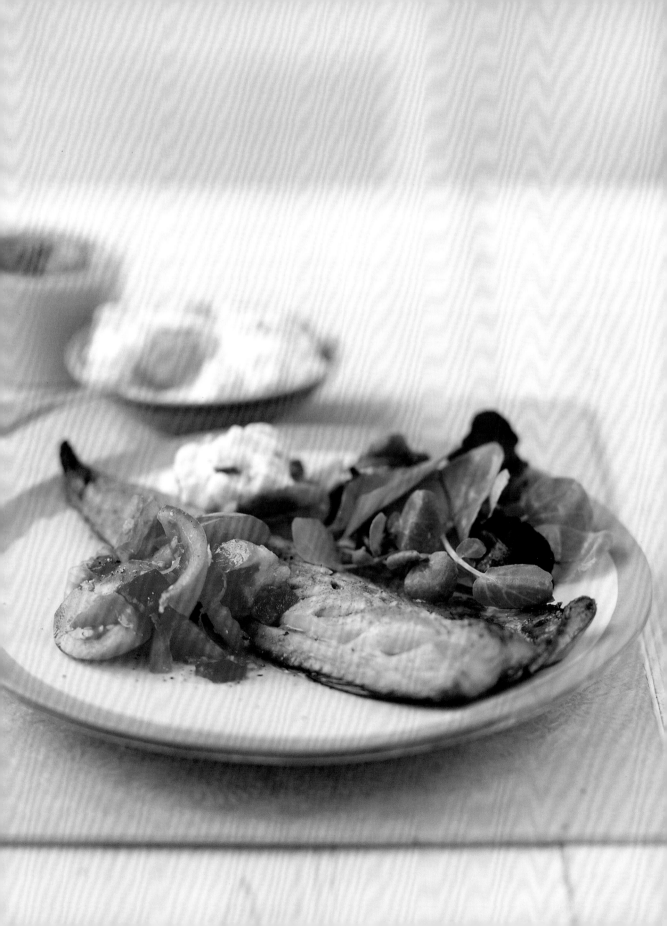

chimichurri steak

Argentinian chimichurri sauce provides the perfect acidity and freshness for steak.

Ingredients

2 rump steaks, 240 g (8½ oz) each, trimmed of fat

4 medium tomatoes, sliced in half

4 tsp olive oil

1 clove garlic, crushed

4 spring onions, finely sliced

flat-leaf parsley leaves, handful, roughly chopped

coriander leaves, handful, roughly chopped

2 tsp red wine vinegar

½ lime, juice

1–2 green chillies (depending on taste), finely chopped

salad leaves

black pepper

Method

1 Remove the steaks from the fridge and allow to come up to cool room temperature. Preheat a griddle pan or heavy frying pan over a medium–high heat.

2 Rub the steaks and the tomatoes in 2 teaspoons of the oil and cook the steaks on the griddle for 2 minutes on each side for medium-rare, 3 minutes for medium or 4 minutes for well done.

3 Add the tomatoes, cut-side down, for the final 3 minutes of cooking. Remove the steaks and tomatoes from the pan and allow to rest for 10 minutes.

4 Meanwhile, make the chimichurri sauce by combining the remaining oil with the garlic, spring onions, herbs, vinegar, lime juice and chillies. Add black pepper, to taste.

5 Slice the steaks and divide into 4. Serve with a large spoonful of chimichurri sauce, tomatoes and salad leaves.

Tips & variations

For a vegetarian alternative use 160 g (5½ oz) each of asparagus, sliced aubergine and courgette and grill with the tomato (this provides 0 servings of protein and 3 servings of vegetables).

SERVINGS		NUTRITION	
0	Carbohydrates	202	Calories
4	Protein	4 g	Carbohydrates
½	Fat	28 g	Protein
0	Dairy	2 g	Fibre
1½	Vegetables	0.2 g	Salt
0	Fruit		

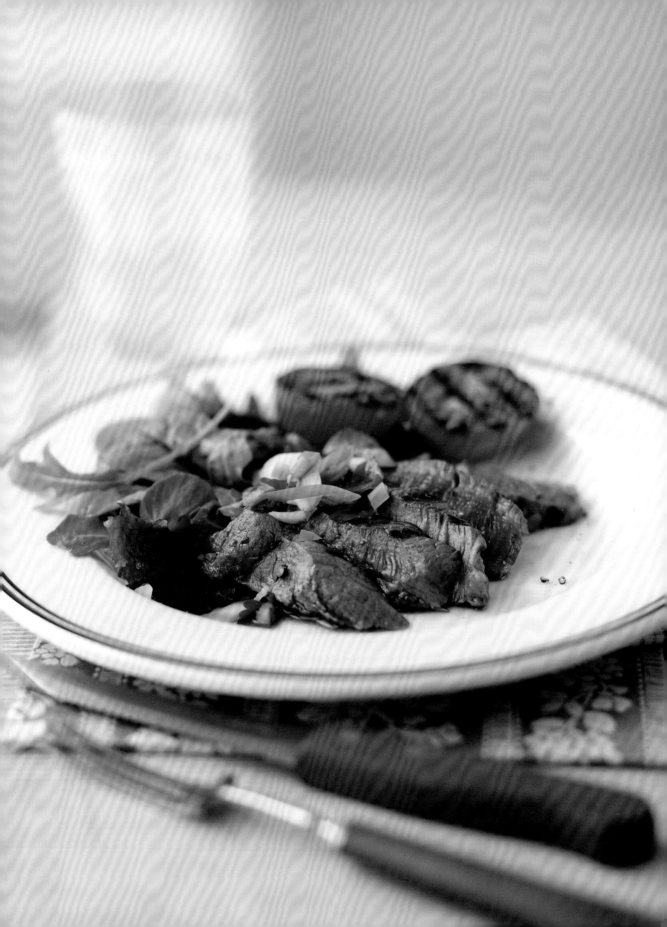

Thai beef salad

This aromatic salad combines sharp citrus with fiery heat and cool, crisp flavours.

Ingredients

2.5-cm (1-in) piece ginger, peeled and finely grated

1 stick lemon grass, finely sliced (woody outer leaves removed)

1 tbsp fish sauce

1 tsp low-salt soy sauce

2 tsp sesame oil

1 lime, juice

1 red chilli, finely chopped (de-seeded if liked)

2 rump steaks, 240 g (8½ oz) each, trimmed of fat

100 g (3½ oz) salad leaves

10-cm (4-in) piece cucumber, cut into spears

80 g (2¾ oz) cherry tomatoes, cut into quarters

80 g (2¾ oz) bean sprouts

coriander, basil and mint leaves, small handful of each, roughly torn

Method

1 Mix together the ginger, lemon grass, fish sauce, soy sauce, sesame oil, lime juice and chilli. Pour one half of the marinade over the steak and reserve the other half. Allow the steak to marinate for a minimum of 10 minutes or overnight.

2 Preheat the grill to high. Remove the steaks from the marinade and grill for 2 minutes on each side for medium-rare, 3 minutes for medium or 4 minutes for well done. Remove the steaks from under the grill and set aside to rest for 10 minutes before slicing.

3 Toss the steak in the reserved marinade and add the remaining ingredients. Toss to coat before serving.

Tips & variations

The marinade makes a great dressing and is good to have on hand to add vibrancy to a salad. For a vegetarian alternative use a packet of firm tofu (approximately 400 g/14 oz) sliced into 4, marinate in the same way, using more soy sauce instead of the fish sauce, and grill for 2 minutes each side (2 servings protein).

SERVINGS		NUTRITION	
0	Carbohydrates	192	Calories
4	Protein	3 g	Carbohydrates
0	Fat	28 g	Protein
0	Dairy	2 g	Fibre
1½	Vegetables	0.3 g	Salt
0	Fruit		

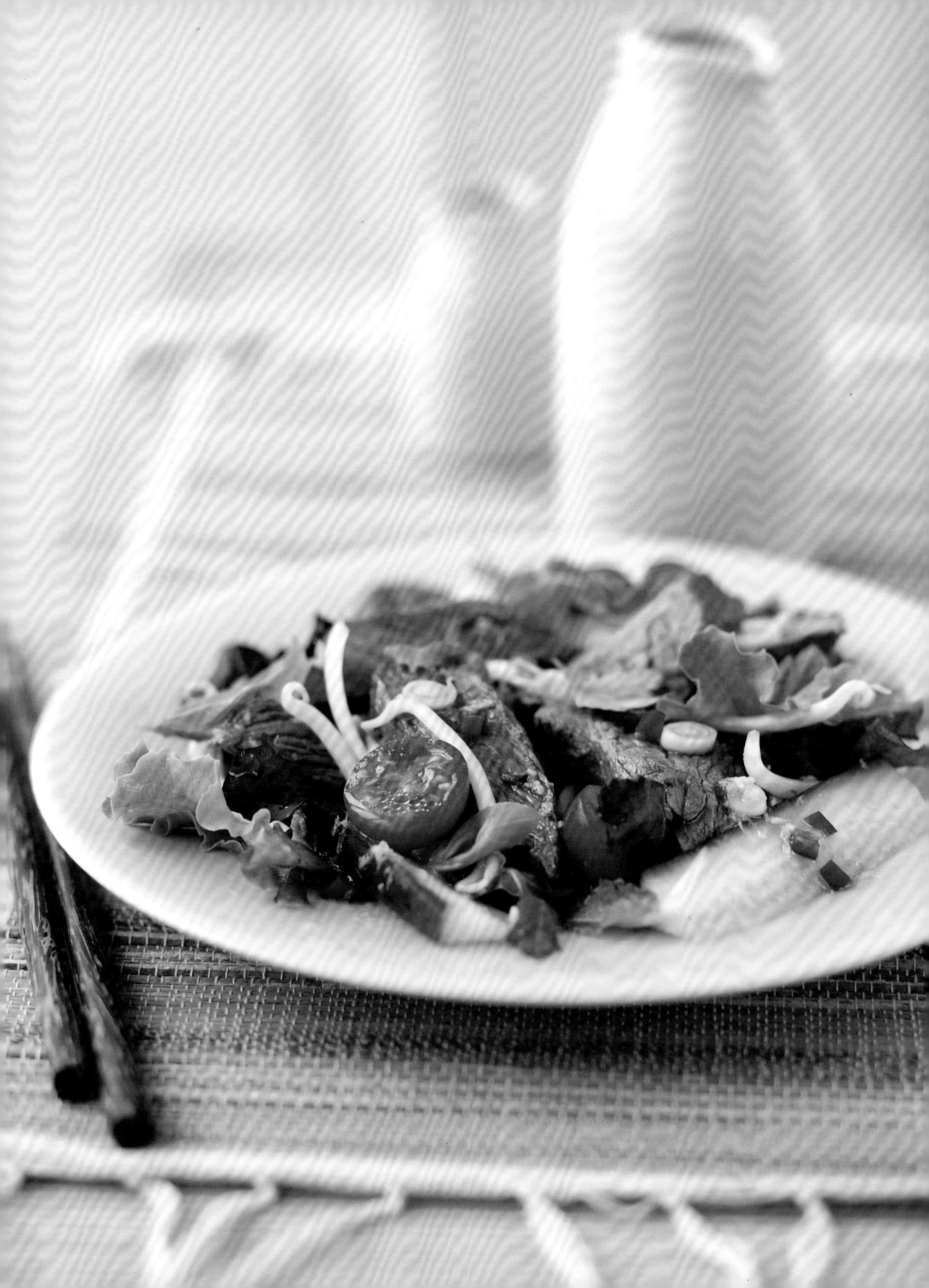

lamb steaks with rocket & mint salsa & kale

Lamb steaks are the ideal choice for a quick and easy meal.

Ingredients

4 lamb leg steaks, trimmed of fat, approximately 120 g (4 oz) each

3 tsp olive oil

1 clove garlic, crushed

160 g (5½ oz) rocket leaves, roughly chopped

mint leaves, large handful, roughly chopped

160 g (5½ oz) cherry tomatoes, sliced in half

1 tbsp capers, drained and roughly chopped

1½ tbsp red wine vinegar

320 g (11 oz) curly kale, tough central stalk cut out, finely chopped

black pepper

Method

1 Remove the lamb from the fridge and allow to come up to cool room temperature. Preheat the grill to high.

2 Rub the lamb with 1 teaspoon of the oil and season with pepper. Grill for 2–3 minutes on each side for medium, 4 minutes on each side for well done. Allow to rest for 10 minutes.

3 Meanwhile, make the salsa by stirring together the remaining oil, the garlic, rocket, mint, tomatoes, capers and vinegar. Season, to taste, with black pepper.

4 Blanch the kale in boiling water for 2 minutes. Serve the lamb on a bed of kale with the salsa spooned over the steak.

Tips & variations

You can use watercress instead of rocket if you prefer the flavour. Lamb steaks also work well with a garlic and rosemary marinade – serve with couscous on an unrestricted day.

SERVINGS		NUTRITION	
0	Carbohydrates	249	Calories
4	Protein	4 g	Carbohydrates
0	Fat	29 g	Protein
0	Dairy	3 g	Fibre
2	Vegetables	0.4 g	Salt
0	Fruit		

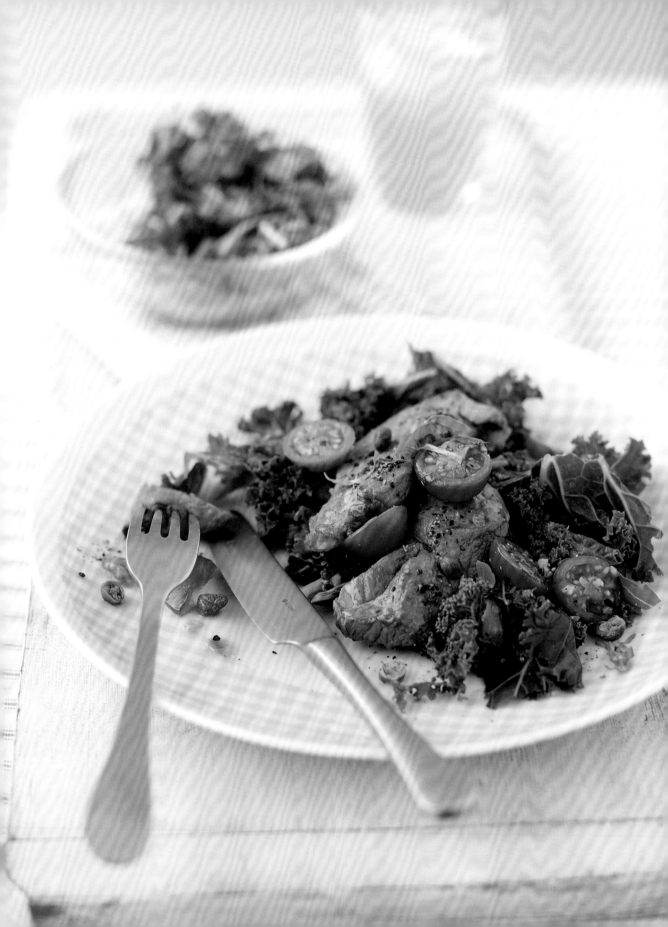

herb & mustard-crusted pork fillet with Mediterranean vegetables

This one-pan dish makes for a hearty, healthy meal and is a cinch to prepare.

Ingredients

480 g (1 lb 1 oz) pork tenderloin, halved

1 tbsp sage leaves, finely chopped

1 tbsp thyme leaves, finely chopped

1 tbsp parsley leaves, finely chopped

2 tbsp wholegrain mustard

3 tsp olive oil

½ lemon, juice and zest

1 medium aubergine, cut into 1-cm (½-in) slices

1 large courgette, cut into 1-cm (½-in) slices

320 g (11 oz) cherry tomatoes

2 cloves garlic, crushed

2 tsp balsamic vinegar

black pepper

Method

1 Preheat the oven to 200°C/400°F/gas mark 6. Lay the pork fillets on a board. In a small bowl combine the herbs, mustard, 1 teaspoon of the oil and half of the lemon juice and zest. Season with black pepper. Spread this mixture evenly over the fillets and transfer to a large baking tray.

2 Toss the vegetables and tomatoes in the remaining lemon juice and zest, oil, garlic and vinegar and lay them around the pork fillets. Transfer to the oven and cook for 20–25 minutes, until the pork is completely cooked through.

3 Once out of the oven, allow the meat to rest for 5–10 minutes (keep the vegetables warm) before slicing. Divide equally into 4 and serve.

Tips & variations

For an intense flavour, marinate the pork overnight after rubbing in the herbs, mustard, oil and lemon juice. If you don't like mustard try adding finely chopped dried apricots for a fruity alternative.

SERVINGS		NUTRITION	
0	Carbohydrates	217	Calories
4	Protein	6 g	Carbohydrates
0	Fat	30 g	Protein
0	Dairy	4 g	Fibre
2½	Vegetables	0.8 g	Salt
0	Fruit		

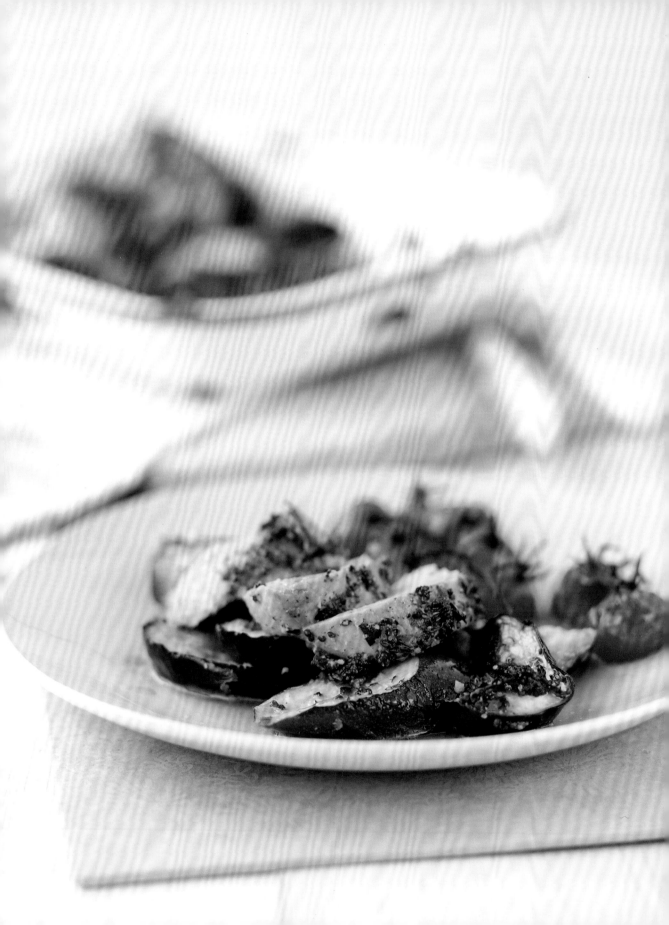

Moroccan-spiced pork fillet

with fennel & preserved lemon

Ras-el-hanout is a classic Moroccan spice mix available in most supermarkets.

Ingredients

480 g (1 lb 1 oz) pork tenderloin, halved

3 tsp olive oil

1 tbsp ras-el-hanout

320 g (11 oz) fennel, finely sliced

160 g (5½ oz) salad leaves

½ tsp sumac or the zest of 1 lemon, finely grated

1 preserved lemon, cut into quarters, flesh cut away and discarded, zest finely sliced

1 tbsp mint leaves, roughly torn

1 tbsp flat-leaf parsley, roughly chopped

Method

1 Preheat the oven to 200°C/400°F/gas mark 6. Rub the pork with 1 teaspoon of the oil and the ras-el-hanout.

2 Toss the fennel in the remaining oil and transfer to a large baking tray. Lay the pork on top of the fennel and transfer to the oven. Cook for 20–25 minutes, turning the pork and fennel over halfway through cooking, until the pork is cooked through.

3 Remove the pork from the tray, allow to rest for 5–10 minutes before slicing.

4 Serve the pork slices on a bed of fennel with green salad on the side. Sprinkle with the sumac, preserved lemon, mint and parsley.

Tips & variations

If you can't find ras-el-hanout, replace it with 1 tablespoon of Moroccan spices or mix together ¼ tsp ground turmeric, ¼ tsp ground ginger, ½ tsp ground cinnamon, ½ tsp ground cumin and ½ tsp paprika. If you can't find preserved lemons, use an ordinary fresh lemon instead.

SERVINGS		NUTRITION	
0	Carbohydrates	177	Calories
4	Protein	2 g	Carbohydrates
0	Fat	28 g	Protein
0	Dairy	3 g	Fibre
1½	Vegetables	0.2 g	Salt
0	Fruit		

venison & blackberries

with a celeriac & rocket mash

Blackberries bring freshness to the rich, earthy venison in this sophisticated dish.

Ingredients

4 tsp olive oil

4 venison steaks, approximately 120 g (4 oz) each, trimmed of fat

500 ml (17 fl oz) low-salt chicken stock

320 g (11 oz) celeriac, peeled and roughly chopped

1 clove garlic, crushed

200 ml (7 fl oz) low-salt beef stock

1 tbsp balsamic vinegar

1 tsp thyme leaves, roughly chopped

160 g (5½ oz) blackberries

1 tbsp flat-leaf parsley, roughly chopped

80 g (2¾ oz) rocket leaves

black pepper

Method

1 Heat 1 teaspoon of the oil in a frying pan over a medium heat. Add the venison and cook for 5 minutes, then turn over and cook for a further 3–5 minutes for medium. Cook for 5–6 minutes on each side for well done. Remove from the pan and set aside to rest.

2 Meanwhile, bring the chicken stock to the boil in a large saucepan and add the celeriac. Simmer for 10 minutes, until the celeriac is soft, then drain.

3 To make the sauce, place the venison pan back on the heat and add the garlic. Fry for 30 seconds before adding the beef stock and vinegar. Simmer for 2–3 minutes until slightly reduced before adding the thyme and blackberries. Simmer for a further 2 minutes, until the blackberries have softened slightly.

4 Mash the celeriac with the remaining oil. Season with black pepper and stir through the parsley and rocket. Serve alongside the venison steak with the sauce poured over the top.

Tips & variations

If you want to use a different type of meat, try lamb.

SERVINGS		NUTRITION	
0	Carbohydrates	192	Calories
4	Protein	5 g	Carbohydrates
½	Fat	30 g	Protein
0	Dairy	4 g	Fibre
1½	Vegetables	1.3 g	Salt
½	Fruit		

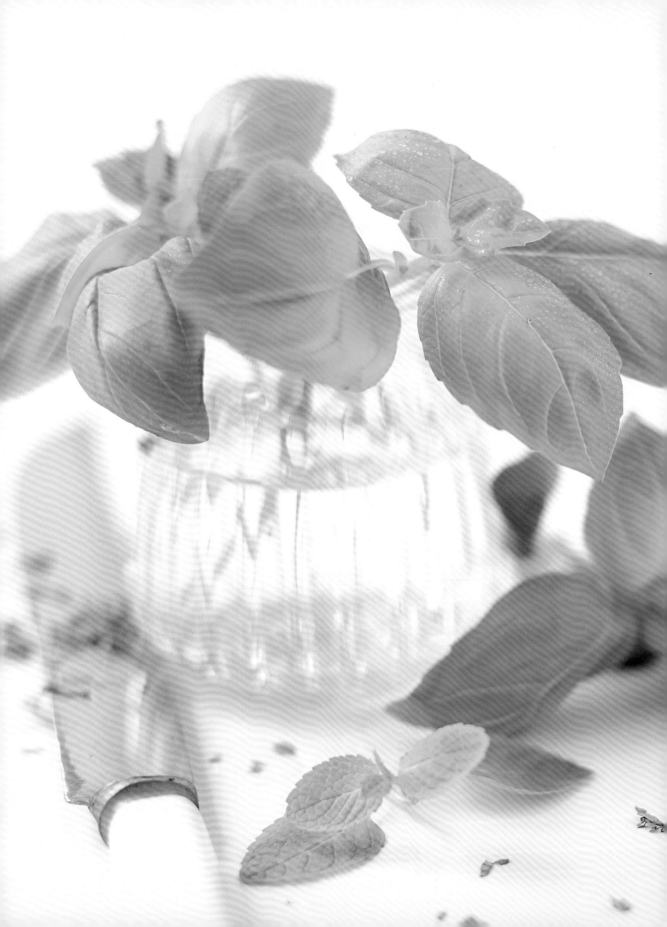

restricted days
quick & easy
vegetarian mains

Middle-Eastern kale salad

The Middle-Eastern spice mix, za'atar, is at the heart of this wholesome, comforting dish.

Ingredients

1 tbsp sumac or the zest of 1 lemon, finely grated

1 tbsp dried thyme

2 tsp toasted sesame seeds

1 tsp dried marjoram

1 tsp dried oregano

320 g (11 oz) kale, central stalk removed, shredded

1 tbsp lemon juice

300 g (10½ oz) low-fat Greek yoghurt

4 tbsp mint leaves, roughly torn

8 eggs

black pepper

Method

1 To make the za'atar, combine the sumac or lemon zest, thyme, sesame seeds, marjoram and oregano and either pound the mixture lightly with a pestle and mortar or grind in a spice grinder until fine, with a little texture.

2 Blanch the kale in boiling water for 1–2 minutes, until just softened. Drain well and transfer to a bowl. Sprinkle over the za'atar and lemon juice and stir to combine. Stir the yoghurt and mint together in a separate bowl.

3 To poach the eggs, bring a large pan of water to the boil and crack 2 eggs into it. Turn the heat down and simmer for 4 minutes; repeat with the 6 remaining eggs. Drain well.

4 Lay the eggs on a bed of kale and serve with the yoghurt and mint on the side. Sprinkle with black pepper.

Tips & variations

Za'atar is an extremely versatile spice mix that you can scatter over vegetables before you roast them. Alternatively sprinkle it over salads for extra flavour. You can use ordinary plain yoghurt (whole-milk or low-fat) or low-fat fromage frais instead of low-fat Greek yoghurt if you prefer.

SERVINGS		NUTRITION	
0	Carbohydrates	277	Calories
2	Protein	7 g	Carbohydrates
0	Fat	23 g	Protein
½	Dairy	2 g	Fibre
1	Vegetables	0.7 g	Salt
0	Fruit		

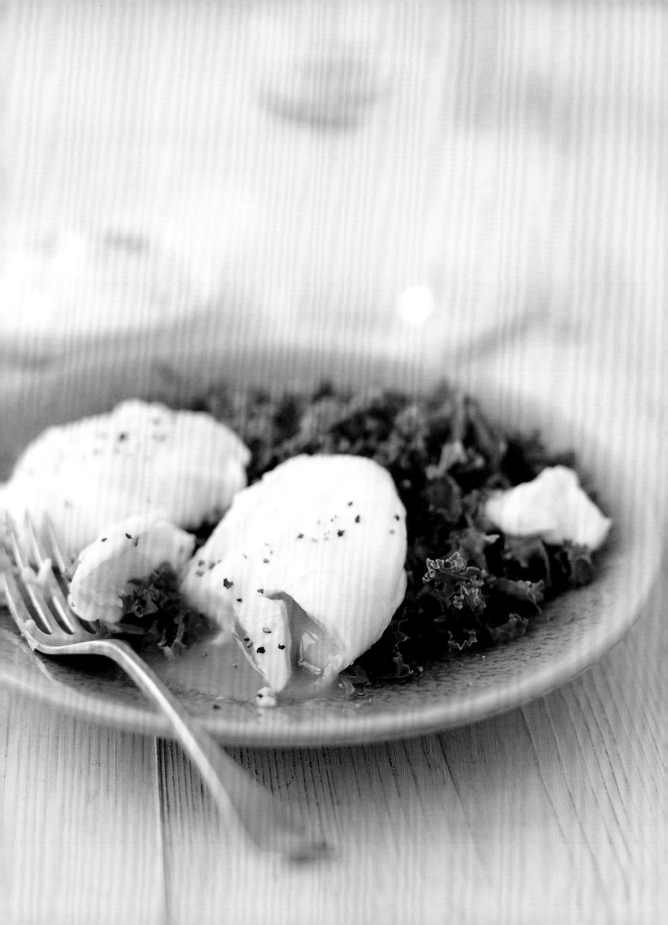

okra & tomato curry with paneer

Paneer cheese and delicate okra provide the perfect basis for this spicy vegetarian dish.

Ingredients

3 tsp rapeseed oil

2.5-cm (1-in) piece ginger, peeled and finely grated

3 cloves garlic, crushed

2 tsp ground cumin

2 tsp ground coriander

1 tsp ground turmeric

180 g (6⅓ oz) paneer cheese, cubed

2 x 400-g (14-oz) tins tomatoes, chopped

320 g (11 oz) okra

1½ tsp garam masala

coriander leaves, small handful, to serve

1 lemon, cut into wedges

Method

1 Heat the oil in a large frying pan over a medium heat. Add the ginger, garlic, cumin, coriander and turmeric and cook for 30 seconds, until fragrant.

2 Add the paneer and cook for 3–4 minutes, until golden brown on all sides. Remove from the pan and set aside.

3 Add the tomatoes to the pan and simmer for 5–8 minutes (adding 100 ml/3½ fl oz water to avoid them drying out), until slightly reduced, before adding the paneer and the okra.

4 Simmer for 5 minutes, sprinkle over the garam masala and serve with coriander and lemon wedges.

Tips & variations

Although paneer is absolutely delicious cooked, try it raw, tossed into salads for a quick vegetarian lunch. Make sure you choose paneer cheese made with semi-skimmed milk.

SERVINGS		NUTRITION	
0	Carbohydrates	145	Calories
0	Protein	10 g	Carbohydrates
0	Fat	9 g	Protein
1½	Dairy	5 g	Fibre
2	Vegetables	0.3 g	Salt
0	Fruit		

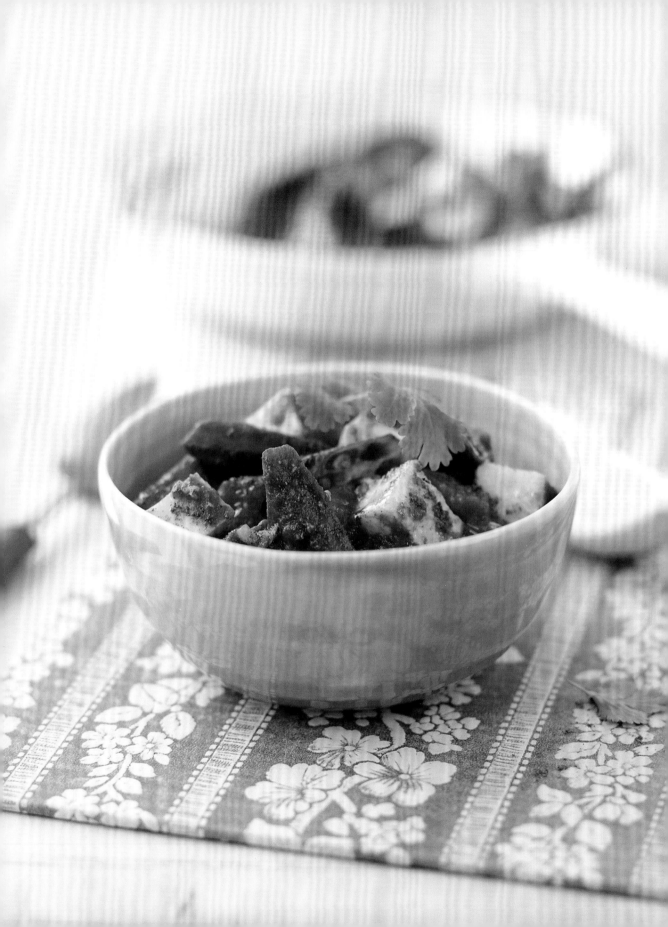

smoked aubergine salad

This salad combines the rich, smoky flavours of baba ganoush.

Ingredients

3 small aubergines, combined weight approximately 480 g (1 lb 1 oz)

120 g (4 oz) green beans, trimmed

240 g (8½ oz) soya beans, thawed if frozen

12 spring onions, finely sliced

240 g (8½ oz) cherry tomatoes, sliced in half

1 lemon, juice

3 tsp olive oil

2 tbsp mint leaves, roughly torn

flat-leaf parsley leaves, large handful

2 tsp sumac or zest of 1 lemon, finely grated

Method

1 Preheat a griddle pan to high. When smoking hot, add the aubergines and griddle for 10–15 minutes, until blistered and charred. Remove from the pan and set aside, cover in cling film.

2 Meanwhile, blanch the green beans and soya beans in boiling water for 2 minutes. Drain and run under cold water to refresh.

3 Peel the charred skin away from the aubergine and roughly chop the flesh. Toss with the beans, spring onions, tomatoes, lemon juice, oil, herbs and sumac or lemon zest.

Tips & variations

To save time, you can char the aubergines the day before you need it and keep it in the fridge overnight.

SERVINGS		NUTRITION	
0	Carbohydrates	146	Calories
2	Protein	10 g	Carbohydrates
0	Fat	11 g	Protein
0	Dairy	9 g	Fibre
3	Vegetables	<0.1 g	Salt
0	Fruit		

soya bean burger with a nut coating

Burgers may sound a little 'off-diet', but these are super-healthy and packed with protein.

Ingredients

240 g (8½ oz) soya beans, thawed if frozen and blanched in boiling water for 3 minutes

30 g (1 oz) low-fat mozzarella, finely chopped

1 egg, beaten

1 tsp flat-leaf parsley leaves, finely chopped

1 tsp coriander leaves

1 red chilli, de-seeded, roughly chopped

4 spring onions, sliced

120 g (4 oz) whole almonds

320 g (11 oz) Little Gem lettuce leaves

320 g (11 oz) cherry tomatoes, chopped

1 lime, juice

Method

1 To make the burgers, put the beans, mozzarella, egg, parsley, coriander, chilli and spring onions in a food processor and pulse until the mixture resembles a paste. The mixture should hold together well, so if it looks crumbly add a tablespoonful of water.

2 Divide the mixture into 8 and form patties. Meanwhile, clean the food processor and blitz the almonds until finely chopped, but not too fine and powdery. Dip the patties in the almonds until covered and refrigerate for 30 minutes.

3 Preheat the oven to 200°C/400°F/gas mark 6. Place the burgers on a lightly oiled baking tray. Bake in the oven for 15–20 minutes, until the crusts are golden and the burgers are piping hot.

4 To serve, lay 2 burgers per person on a bed on lettuce leaves, top with the cherry tomatoes and drizzle over the lime juice.

Tips & variations

Use frozen soya beans rather than dried for this recipe – they are quicker to work with, full of nutrients and give the burgers a beautiful, vibrant green colour.

SERVINGS		NUTRITION	
0	Carbohydrates	335	Calories
2	Protein	10 g	Carbohydrates
3½	Fat	20 g	Protein
0	Dairy	9 g	Fibre
2	Vegetables	0.1 g	Salt
0	Fruit		

stuffed courgettes

with feta & sun-dried tomatoes

Pep up courgettes with sharp feta cheese and sundried tomatoes.

Ingredients

- 2 large courgettes, cut in half lengthways, seeds scooped out
- 2 tsp olive oil
- 2 tsp flaked almonds, toasted
- 120 g (4 oz) feta cheese, crumbled
- 8 sun-dried tomatoes, chopped
- 4 spring onions, sliced
- 1 tsp thyme leaves, roughly chopped
- basil leaves, small handful
- 120 g (4 oz) salad leaves
- black pepper

Method

1 Preheat the oven to 220°C/425°F/gas mark 7. Place the courgettes, cut side up, on a baking tray. Brush with half the oil and season with black pepper. Bake in the oven for 15 minutes, until the edges are golden.

2 Mix together the remaining oil, almonds, feta, sun-dried tomatoes, spring onions and thyme leaves and season with black pepper.

3 Sprinkle the filling mix over the courgettes and return to the oven for a further 10 minutes, until golden. Serve with torn basil leaves and salad leaves.

Tips & variations

To save time, make up the stuffing the day before and store it in the fridge overnight.

SERVINGS		NUTRITION	
0	Carbohydrates	144	Calories
0	Protein	3 g	Carbohydrates
½	Fat	7 g	Protein
1	Dairy	2 g	Fibre
1½	Vegetables	1.2 g	Salt
0	Fruit		

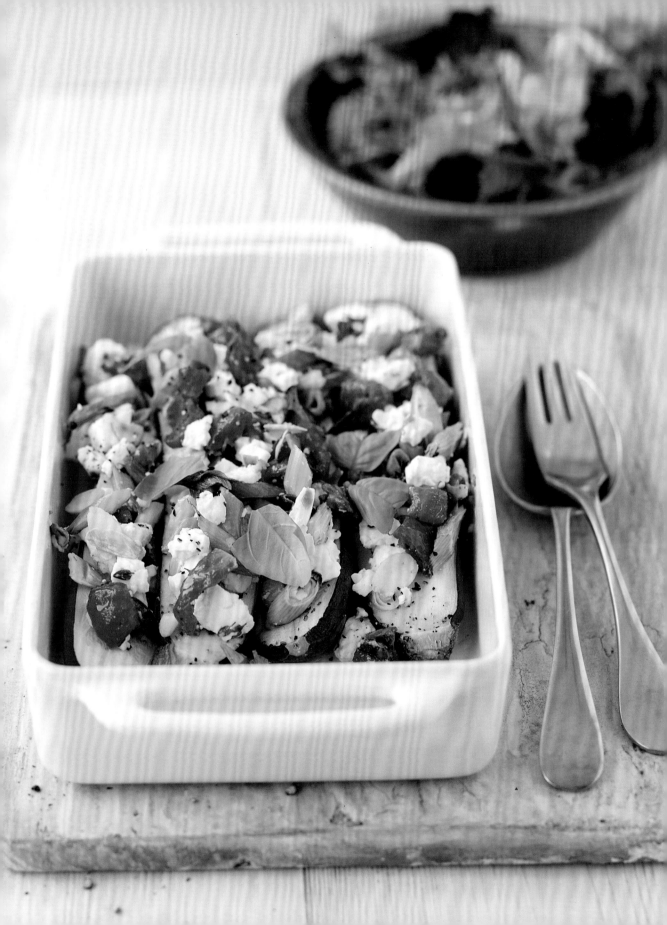

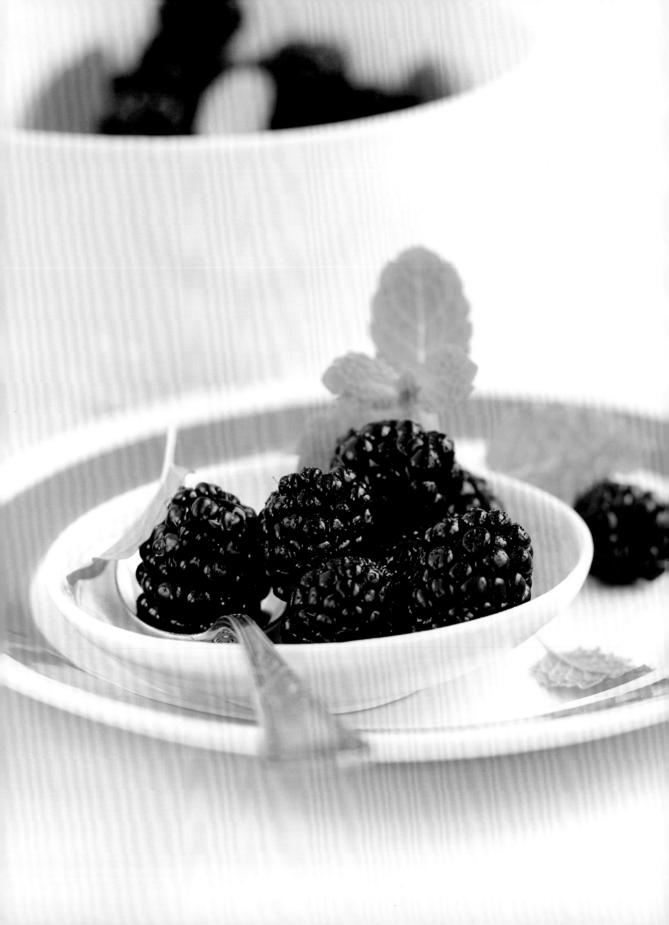

restricted days
desserts

instant blackberry frozen yoghurt

This easy-to-prepare dessert feels like a real treat and it's full of vitamins.

Ingredients

300 g (10½ oz) low-fat Greek yoghurt, frozen

320 g (11 oz) blackberries, setting aside 8 to serve

Method

1 Remove the yoghurt from the freezer and allow it to thaw slightly at room temperature for a few minutes.

2 Whizz the yoghurt and blackberries in a food processor until the mixture is thick and creamy.

3 Serve straight away, with 2 whole blackberries per portion to decorate.

Tips & variations

You can use ordinary plain yoghurt (whole-milk or low-fat) or low-fat fromage frais instead of low-fat Greek yoghurt, if you prefer

SERVINGS		NUTRITION	
0	Carbohydrates	79	Calories
0	Protein	10 g	Carbohydrates
0	Fat	5 g	Protein
½	Dairy	4 g	Fibre
0	Vegetables	0.2 g	Salt
1	Fruit		

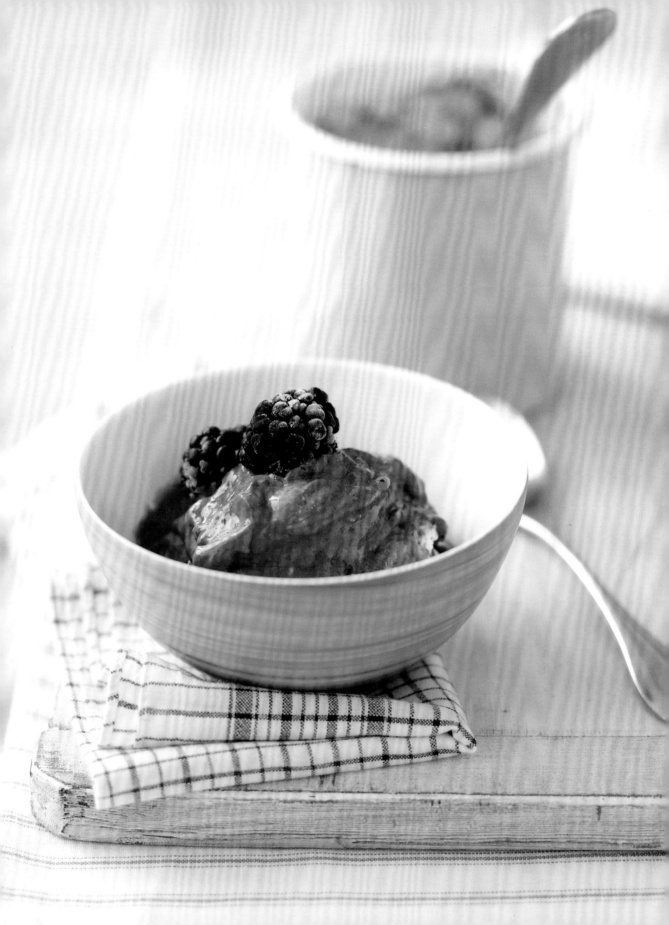

melon, mint & pineapple granita

This delicious, refreshing dessert is perfect for a dinner party and it's as light as a feather.

Ingredients

160 g (5½ oz) cantaloupe melon flesh, roughly chopped

160 g (5½ oz) pineapple flesh, roughly chopped

2 tbsp mint leaves

Method

1 Put the melon, pineapple and mint in a food processor and blitz until liquefied. Transfer to a punnet or freezer-proof container and stir in 150 ml (5 fl oz) water.

2 Freeze for 20 minutes until ice crystals start to form. Remove from the freezer and use a fork to break up the crystals. Return to the freezer until firm.

3 Transfer to the fridge for 30 minutes before serving.

Tips & variations

Add a teaspoon of freshly grated ginger to create a wonderfully fiery dessert.

SERVINGS		NUTRITION	
0	Carbohydrates	14	Calories
0	Protein	3 g	Carbohydrates
0	Fat	0 g	Protein
0	Dairy	1 g	Fibre
0	Vegetables	<0.1 g	Salt
1	Fruit		

For a picture of this recipe see page 2.

rhubarb fool

This is a lighter version of the comforting childhood classic.

Ingredients

300 g (10½ oz) low-fat Greek yoghurt

320 g (11 oz) rhubarb, stewed with a little water and sweetener (granulated, non-calorie)

4 tsp toasted seeds

Method

1 Spoon a little of the yoghurt into 4 bowls or shallow glasses, followed by a little rhubarb.

2 Continue to layer up until the yoghurt and rhubarb are used up. Sprinkle over the seeds and serve.

Tips & variations

Stewed rhubarb is great to have on standby in the freezer – you can use it as a base for a quick dessert. You can also use ordinary plain yoghurt (whole-milk or low-fat) or low-fat fromage frais instead of low-fat Greek yoghurt if you prefer.

SERVINGS		NUTRITION	
0	Carbohydrates	88	Calories
0	Protein	7 g	Carbohydrates
½	Fat	6 g	Protein
½	Dairy	2 g	Fibre
0	Vegetables	0.2 g	Salt
1	Fruit		

part 2 unrestricted days

recipes

V indicates that the recipe is suitable for vegetarians; **VT** indicates vegetarian tip – that the recipe includes advice on adapting it for vegetarians.

SNACK IDEAS/UNRESTRICTED DAYS

- oatcakes, rye crispbreads or wholemeal crackers with low-fat hummus, low-fat cheese or cottage cheese
- fruit
- vegetable crudités such as celery, cucumber, green peppers, mangetout, spring onions and cherry tomatoes with salsa, low-fat hummus, tzatziki or guacamole
- yoghurt
- malt loaf with or without margarine or low-fat spread
- small handful of unsalted nuts (for example, walnuts, pistachio nuts or Brazil nuts) or dried fruit (for example, apricots, figs, sultanas or mango)
- a glass of vegetable juice (carrot, tomato or a mixture)
- plain popcorn (popped in vegetable oil with no sugar or salt added)
- bowl of soup
- smoothie made with skimmed or semi-skimmed milk, yoghurt and one piece of fruit
- dried pea snacks
- sugar-free jelly
- ice lolly made from frozen, diluted, sugar-free fruit cordial

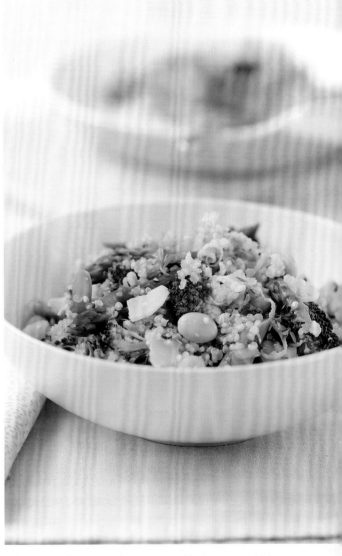

Lemon-scented quinoa and spring vegetable risotto, page 124

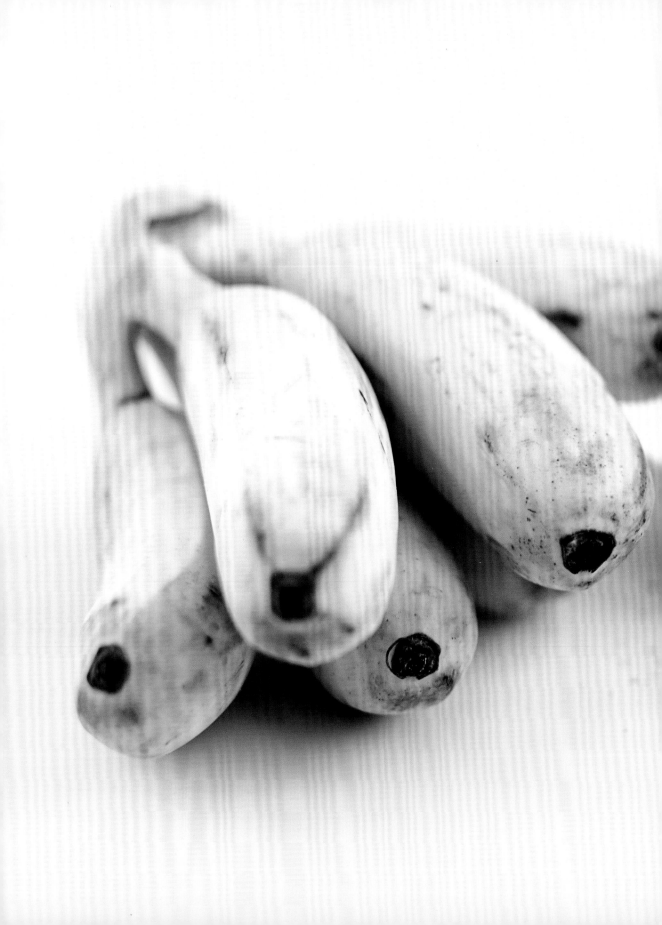

unrestricted days
breakfasts

wholemeal banana & flaxseed pancakes

These wholesome, comforting pancakes are just the thing for a leisurely breakfast or brunch.

Ingredients

100 g (3½ oz) wholemeal self-raising flour

1 tbsp flaxseeds

1 egg

100 ml (3½ fl oz) semi-skimmed milk

2 small bananas, sliced

2 tsp rapeseed oil

4 tsp runny honey

4 strawberries, hulled and quartered (optional)

Method

1 Sift the flour into a large mixing bowl. Stir in the flaxseeds.

2 Beat together the egg and milk in a jug. Make a well in the centre of the flour mixture and add the egg and milk. Using a whisk, gradually draw the flour into the wet ingredients until smooth. Add the banana and stir through.

3 Heat half the rapeseed oil in a large frying pan over a medium heat and drop in 2 tablespoons of the pancake mix at a time – you should be able to fit 3 pancakes in the pan at once. Fry for 1–2 minutes until golden on the underside and puffed up. Flip over and cook for a further 1–2 minutes.

4 Remove from the pan, keep warm and repeat until the mixture is used up. Serve the pancakes drizzled with the honey and scattered with strawberry pieces (optional).

Tips & variations

The pancakes can be frozen after cooking and re-heated in the toaster for a super-quick breakfast.

SERVINGS		NUTRITION	
1½	Carbohydrates	218	Calories
0	Protein	37 g	Carbohydrates
½	Fat	7 g	Protein
0	Dairy	5 g	Fibre
0	Vegetables	0.1 g	Salt
½	Fruit		

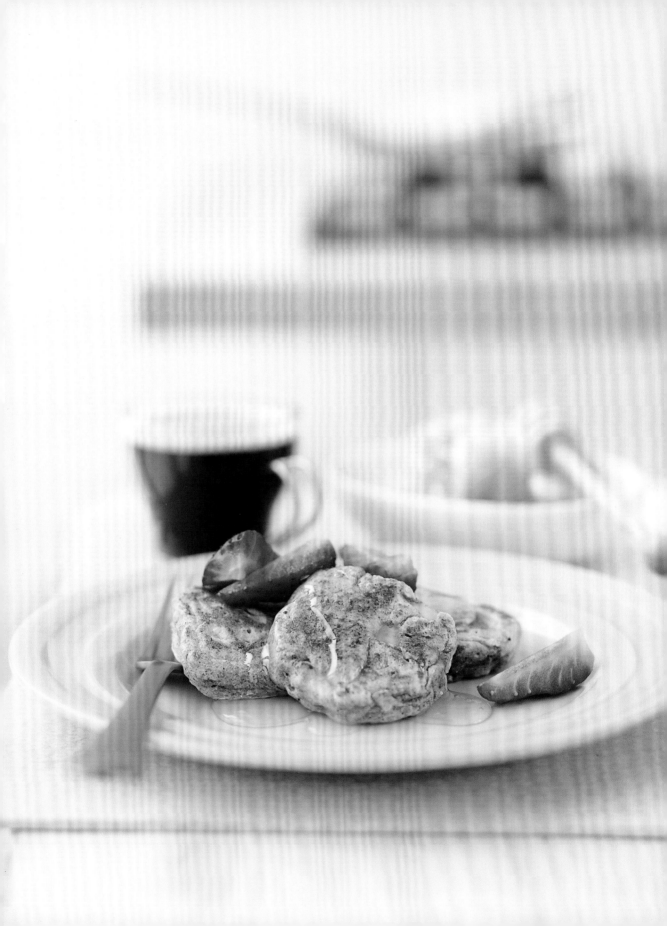

baked ham & egg in a bread cup

These little breakfast cups are so easy to prepare and are absolutely delicious.

Ingredients

1 slice wholemeal bread, crusts removed

½ tsp low-fat spread

20 g (¾ oz) baby spinach leaves

1 medium slice lean ham

1 egg

½ spring onion, finely sliced

15 g (½ oz) low-fat Cheddar, grated

nutmeg, a few grates

black pepper

Tips & variations

The egg can also be paired with cooked leeks, ham and mushrooms, tomatoes, Parmesan and basil – or simply with cheese. For a vegetarian alternative use 1 tbsp of low-fat cream cheese instead of the ham (represents 1 serving of protein and 1½ servings of dairy).

Method

1 Preheat the oven to 180°C/350°F/gas mark 4. Lay the bread out on a board and flatten it thoroughly with a rolling pin to make it thinner. Use the low-fat spread on both sides.

2 Push the slice of bread into a cup in a large muffin tray and fold out the edges to make a flower shape. Bake in the oven for 4–5 minutes, until the bread cup is lightly golden and crisp.

3 Wilt the spinach leaves by rinsing them and then steaming them for 1 minute. Run under cold water and dry thoroughly on kitchen towel.

4 Lay the spinach leaves in the bottom of the bread cup and fold in the ham, pressing down firmly. Crack an egg into the bread cup, leaving a little egg white in the shell if the cup becomes too full. Sprinkle over the spring onions, followed by the cheese and nutmeg. Grind over some black pepper and bake for about 20 minutes until the egg white is just set.

5 Check the egg cup after 10 minutes – if the edges are turning too brown, loosely cover with foil and return to the oven. Run a knife around the tray to release the bread cup and serve immediately.

SERVINGS		NUTRITION	
1	Carbohydrates	257	Calories
1½	Protein	16 g	Carbohydrates
½	Fat	20 g	Protein
½	Dairy	3 g	Fibre
0	Vegetables	1.8 g	Salt
0	Fruit		

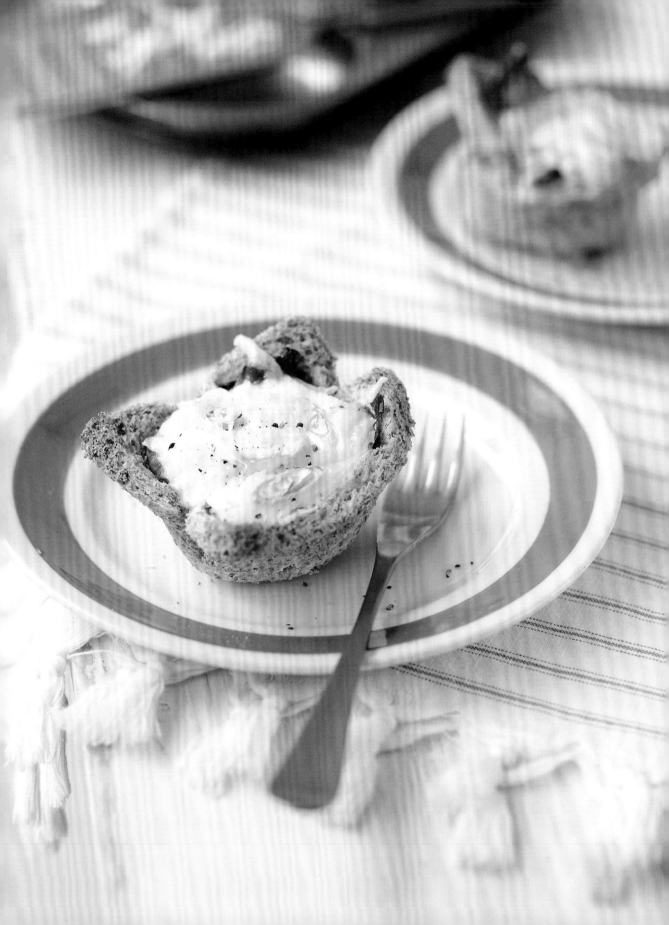

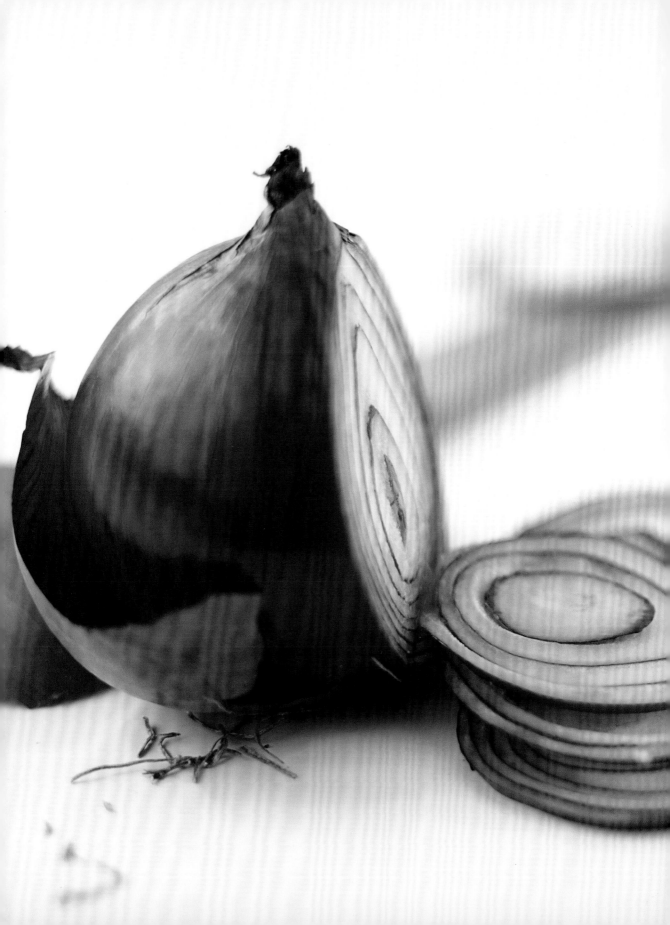

unrestricted days
lunches on the go

herbed quinoa salad

with squash, feta & red onion

This easy-to-prepare lunch is good hot or cold, so it's just the thing to put in your lunchbox.

Ingredients

60 g (2 oz) quinoa

160 g (5½ oz) butternut squash, peeled and cut into 1-cm (½-in) chunks

½ small red onion, sliced

1 clove garlic, crushed

2 tsp olive oil

½ tsp cumin

½ tsp sumac or zest of ½ lemon, finely grated

dried chilli flakes, pinch

30 g (1 oz) feta cheese, crumbled

15 g (½ oz) dried cranberries

2 tsp lemon juice

1 tbsp dill, roughly chopped

1 tbsp flat-leaf parsley, roughly chopped

Method

1 Preheat the oven to 200°C/400°F/gas mark 6. Pour the quinoa on to a baking tray and roast for 5 minutes.

2 Meanwhile, combine the squash, onion and garlic in a bowl and toss with the oil, cumin, sumac or lemon zest and chilli flakes.

3 When the quinoa is out of the oven, transfer to a small saucepan and boil according to packet instructions. Drain if necessary and set aside.

4 Pour the vegetable and spice mix onto the baking tray and roast for 20 minutes, turning halfway through the cooking time. The vegetables should be golden all over.

5 Toss the vegetables and quinoa together and when cool mix in the remaining ingredients.

Tips & variations

Roasting the quinoa before boiling it gives it a lovely nutty flavour. If you're short on time, leave out this step and boil according to the packet instructions.

SERVINGS		NUTRITION	
2	Carbohydrates	430	Calories
0	Protein	61 g	Carbohydrates
1	Fat	16 g	Protein
1	Dairy	3 g	Fibre
2½	Vegetables	1.2 g	Salt
½	Fruit		

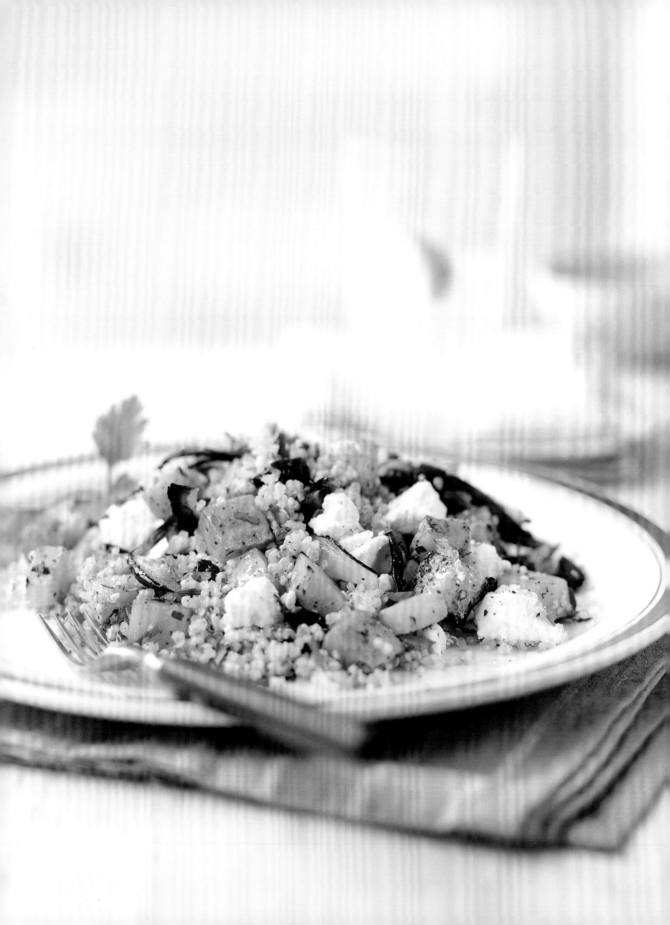

chicken noodle salad

Try this delicious salad – you'll find that the noodles and chilli add Eastern appeal.

Ingredients

350 ml (12 fl oz) low-salt chicken stock

120 g (4 oz) chicken breast

2.5-cm (1-in) piece ginger, peeled and sliced

2 tsp low-salt soy sauce

30 g (1 oz) dried rice noodles

40 g (1½ oz) sugar snap peas, sliced in half

⅓ red pepper, finely sliced

2 spring onions, finely sliced

½ lime, juice

1 tsp fish sauce

1 tsp runny honey

½ red chilli, finely chopped

1 tbsp coriander leaves

1 tbsp mint leaves

1 tbsp basil leaves

1 tbsp toasted unsalted peanuts, roughly chopped

Method

1 Begin by bringing the chicken stock to the boil. Reduce to a simmer and add the chicken, ginger and soy sauce. Cover and simmer for 12–15 minutes, until the chicken is cooked through.

2 Remove the chicken from the stock and set aside to cool. Place the noodles in a bowl. Strain the stock and pour over the noodles. Soak for 4 minutes, or according to the timings on the packet, strain and set aside.

3 Shred the chicken into bite-sized pieces and toss with the noodles, sugar snap peas, red pepper and spring onions. Beat together the lime juice, fish sauce, honey and chilli and pour over the salad. Toss with the remaining ingredients.

Tips & variations

For a vegetarian alternative use 2 eggs instead of the shredded chicken, soy sauce instead of the fish sauce and low-salt vegetable stock instead of the chicken stock. Beat the eggs and fry them in a little oil to make an omelette and then shred (2 protein servings).

SERVINGS		NUTRITION	
1	Carbohydrates	374	Calories
4	Protein	42 g	Carbohydrates
1	Fat	34 g	Protein
0	Dairy	4 g	Fibre
1½	Vegetables	1.1 g	Salt
0	Fruit		

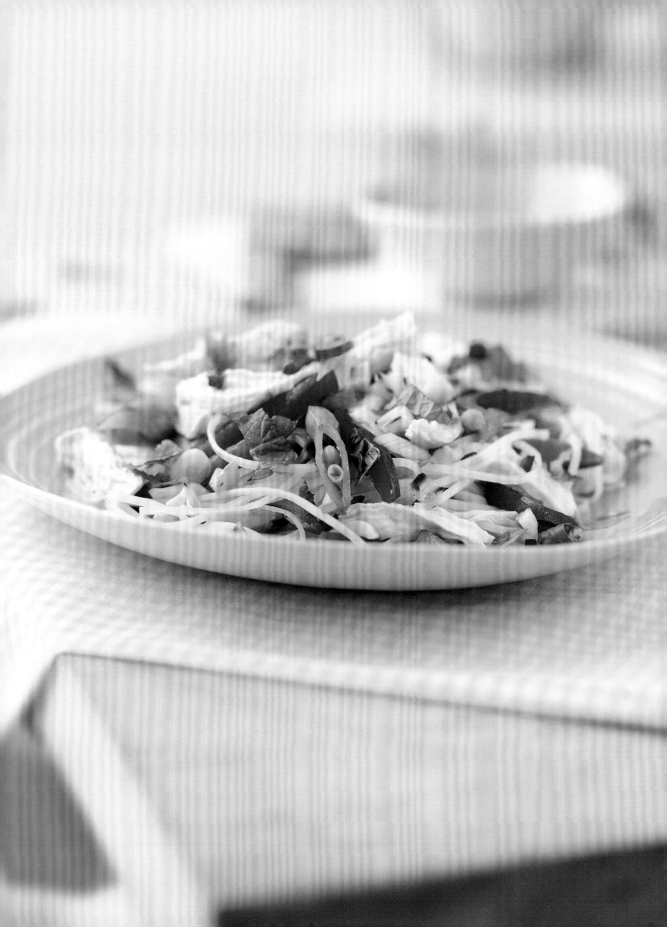

hot-smoked salmon, orange & baby potato salad

So easy to prepare – you can quickly put this salad together the night before, if you like.

Ingredients

120 g (4 oz) baby or new potatoes, halved if large

60 g (2 oz) hot-smoked salmon, flaked into bite-sized pieces

½ orange, cut vertically, skin removed and cut into segments

80 g (2¾ oz) watercress, woody stalks removed

1 tsp red wine vinegar

2 tsp olive oil

1 small shallot, finely sliced

Method

1 Boil the potatoes in a pan of boiling water for 10–15 minutes, until tender. Drain and leave to cool.

2 Toss with the remaining ingredients and serve.

Tips & variations

If you are making this recipe the night before, add the watercress and dressing just before serving to avoid the salad becoming soggy.

SERVINGS		NUTRITION	
1	Carbohydrates	259	Calories
2	Protein	24 g	Carbohydrates
1	Fat	20 g	Protein
0	Dairy	5 g	Fibre
1	Vegetables	3 g	Salt
½	Fruit		

quick mackerel & horseradish pâté with rye crispbread

This super-quick pâté makes for a delicious snack to have on the run.

Ingredients

1 tsp hot horseradish sauce (depending on taste)

1 tbsp low-fat cream cheese

½ tbsp low-fat natural yoghurt

1 tsp lemon juice

45 g (1½ oz) hot-smoked mackerel, skin removed

½ tsp chopped chives

½ tsp dill, finely chopped

2 rye crispbreads

80 g (2½ oz) salad leaves

black pepper

Method

1 Beat together the horseradish and cream cheese, then gradually stir in the yoghurt and lemon juice until smooth.

2 Flake the mackerel and beat into the mixture until it is well mixed but still possessing texture. If the pâté is too thick, add a tablespoon or so of cold water.

3 Season with black pepper, stir through the herbs and serve on the crispbreads with the salad leaves.

Tips & variations

After making, the pâté can be kept in the fridge for up to three days. It can be frozen, but defrost thoroughly in the fridge overnight before serving.

SERVINGS	
1	Carbohydrates
1½	Protein
0	Fat
1	Dairy
1	Vegetables
0	Fruit

NUTRITION	
384	Calories
40 g	Carbohydrates
17 g	Protein
9 g	Fibre
1.3 g	Salt

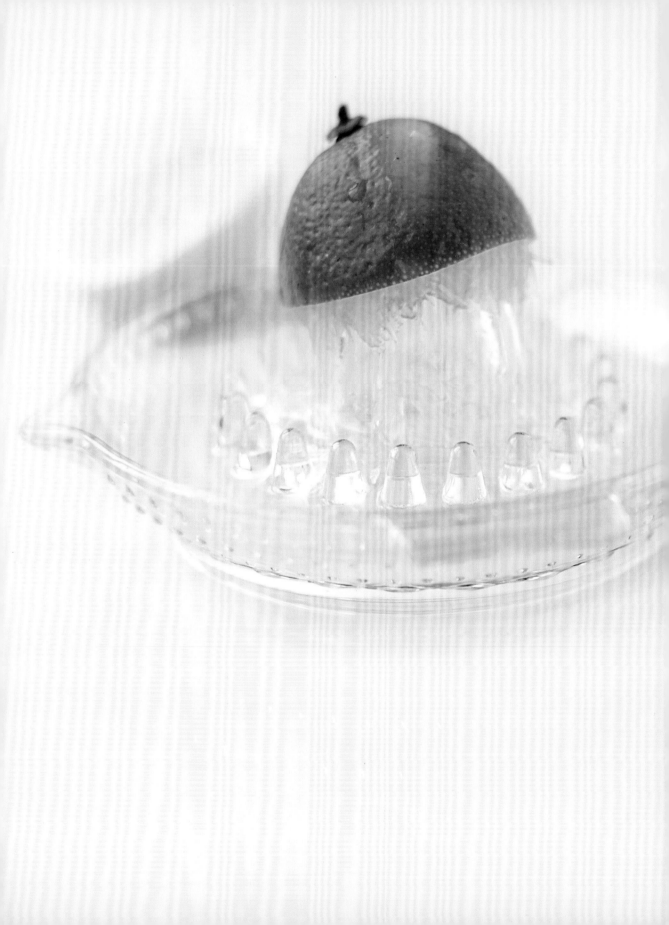

unrestricted days
favourite dinners

turkey, tarragon & mushroom pie with a lemon & herb crust

A healthy take on a classic dish.

Ingredients

2 tsp olive oil

480 g (1 lb 1 oz) turkey breast, cut into bite-sized pieces

2 cloves garlic, crushed

2 medium leeks, finely sliced

1 tsp thyme leaves, roughly chopped

400 ml (13½ fl oz) low-salt chicken stock

160 g (5½ oz) mushrooms

1 tbsp cornflour mixed with 1 tbsp water

4 tbsp low-fat cream cheese

2 tsp Dijon mustard

1 tbsp tarragon, chopped

2 medium slices wholemeal bread, whizzed into breadcrumbs

½ lemon, zest

2 tsp flat-leaf parsley, finely chopped

black pepper

Method

1 Preheat the oven to 200°C/400°F/gas mark 6. Heat 1 teaspoon of the oil in a large saucepan over a medium heat. Add the turkey and garlic and fry for 2–3 minutes, until browned. Remove the turkey from the pan and add the leeks. Cook for a further 2–3 minutes, stirring occasionally.

2 Return the turkey to the pan, add the thyme and stock and bring up to a simmer. Simmer for 5–8 minutes, until the turkey pieces are just cooked through.

3 Strain the stock into a jug and transfer the turkey and leeks to a 1.5 litre (2½ pint) pie dish or 4 individual 400-ml (13-fl oz) pie dishes. Heat the remaining oil in the saucepan and fry the mushrooms for 2–3 minutes, until golden. Transfer to the pie dish or dishes.

4 Pour the stock back into the pan and bring to the boil. Stir in the cornflour mix and stir until the sauce has thickened slightly. Remove from the heat and stir in the cream cheese, mustard and tarragon. Season with a little black pepper and pour into the pie dish, giving the ingredients a good stir.

5 Mix together the breadcrumbs, lemon zest and parsley and scatter over the pie filling. Transfer to the oven and bake for about 15 minutes, or until the breadcrumbs are golden and the sauce bubbling.

SERVINGS		NUTRITION	
1	Carbohydrates	299	Calories
4	Protein	20 g	Carbohydrates
0	Fat	36 g	Protein
1	Dairy	5 g	Fibre
1½	Vegetables	1.1 g	Salt
0	Fruit		

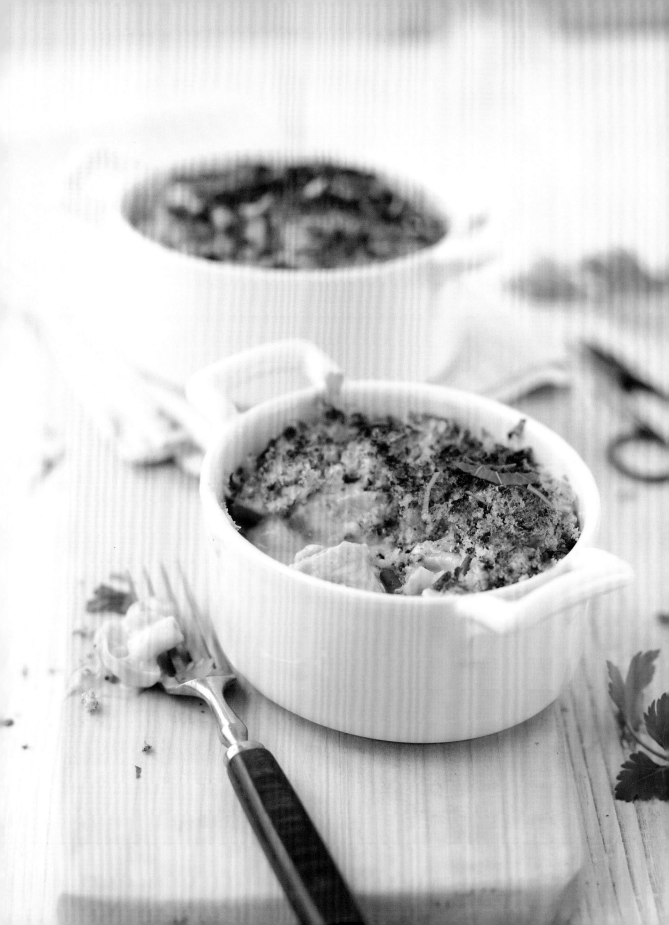

one-pot chicken & veg

Perfect for a lazy Sunday lunch, this tender, aromatic chicken will be a family hit.

Ingredients

1 whole chicken, weighing about 1.5 kg (3 lb)

1 red onion, cut into thick wedges

2 sticks celery, roughly chopped

2 medium leeks, roughly sliced

320 g (11 oz) butternut squash, peeled and cut into large chunks

1 head garlic, halved horizontally

1 lemon, halved

2 bay leaves

thyme sprigs, small handful

2 tsp olive oil

400 ml (14 fl oz) low-salt chicken stock

black pepper

Method

1 Preheat the oven to 200°C/400°F/gas mark 6. Place the chicken in a large roasting tin and scatter the red onion, celery, leeks and butternut squash around it. Tuck half the garlic and lemon inside the bird cavity, plus half the thyme, and tuck the remaining garlic, lemon, bay leave and thyme among the vegetables. Drizzle the oil over the vegetables and bird, season with black pepper and roast for 30 minutes.

2 Remove the chicken from the oven, spoon over the vegetables and baste the chicken in the juices. Lower the oven temperature to 160°C/325°F/gas mark 3 and pour half the stock into the tin and cover the whole of it with foil.

3 Return the tin to the oven for 1¾ hours, until the chicken is cooked through and tender. Remove the chicken from the tin to rest, strain the juices into a small saucepan and keep the vegetables warm.

4 Add the remaining stock to the saucepan and boil for 5 minutes, until reduced. Skim off any fat. Remove the skin and carve. Serve with the vegetables and reduced pan juices.

Tips & variations

The nutrition chart (left) shows information if you skin the chicken before cooking. If you skin it after cooking the nutrition will be 250 calories as the skin adds extra fat. If you remove the skin at the start, keep the chicken covered with foil throughout the cooking time.

SERVINGS		NUTRITION	
0	Carbohydrates	221	Calories
4	Protein	14 g	Carbohydrates
0	Fat	30 g	Protein
0	Dairy	5 g	Fibre
2½	Vegetables	0.3 g	Salt
0	Fruit		

braised french chicken

This delicious one-pot dish is ideal either as a family meal or for a supper party.

Ingredients

2 tsp olive oil

4 free-range skinless chicken breasts, approximately 120 g (4 oz) each

2 rashers lean back bacon, diced

2 cloves garlic, crushed

350 ml (12 fl oz/¾ pint) low-salt chicken stock

4 thyme sprigs

160 g (5½ oz) petits pois

2 Little Gem lettuces, shredded

8 spring onions, sliced

2 tbsp low-fat cream cheese

2 tbsp flat-leaf parsley, roughly chopped

black pepper

Method

1 Heat the oil in a large frying pan. Add the chicken and bacon and fry until golden all over. Add the garlic and continue to fry for a further minute.

2 Pour in the stock, drop in the thyme, lower the heat to a simmer and cover the pan. Simmer the chicken for 12 minutes, until it has just cooked through.

3 Remove the lid and add the petits pois and lettuce. Simmer for 2 minutes and remove from the heat. Stir through the spring onions and cream cheese, season with black pepper and serve sprinkled with parsley.

Tips & variations

This dish can be frozen before the vegetables are added. Defrost the chicken thoroughly in the fridge before using and simmer it in the stock for about 15 minutes (until the chicken is piping hot throughout) before adding the vegetables.

SERVINGS		NUTRITION	
0	Carbohydrates	239	Calories
4½	Protein	5 g	Carbohydrates
0	Fat	35 g	Protein
½	Dairy	4 g	Fibre
1½	Vegetables	1.4 g	Salt
0	Fruit		

roasted cod

with a lemon & breadcrumb crust

A light alternative to fish and chips, this easy supper will satisy any fast-food cravings.

Ingredients

360 g (12½ oz) sweet potatoes, cut into wedges

1 tsp sweet, smoked paprika

4 tsp olive oil

4 cod fillets, about 120 g (4 oz) each

2 medium slices wholemeal bread, whizzed into breadcrumbs

½ lemon, juice and zest

1 tsp thyme leaves, roughly chopped

1 tsp flat-leaf parsley leaves, roughly chopped

320 g (11 oz) green beans, trimmed

1 tbsp mint leaves, roughly chopped

black pepper

Method

1 Preheat the oven to 200°C/400°F/gas mark 6. Begin by mixing the sweet potato wedges with the paprika and 2 teaspoons of the oil. Season with black pepper, transfer to a baking tray and bake in the oven for 10 minutes.

2 Meanwhile, lay the fish on a board and mix together the breadcrumbs, 1 teaspoon of the oil, the lemon zest, the thyme and parsley. Season with black pepper and sprinkle over the cod fillets. Press into the fish to form a crust.

3 Remove the sweet potato wedges from the oven and place the cod fillets among them. Return to the oven for 12–15 minutes, until the fish is just cooked and flakes easily when lightly pressed.

4 Blanch the green beans in boiling water for 3 minutes. Drain and toss with the lemon juice, the remaining oil and the mint.

5 Serve the cod with the beans and sweet potato wedges on the side.

Tips & variations

You can use any firm white fish for this dish such as haddock, coley or pollock.

SERVINGS		NUTRITION	
1½	Carbohydrates	308	Calories
3	Protein	30 g	Carbohydrates
½	Fat	37 g	Protein
0	Dairy	6 g	Fibre
1	Vegetables	0.6 g	Salt
0	Fruit		

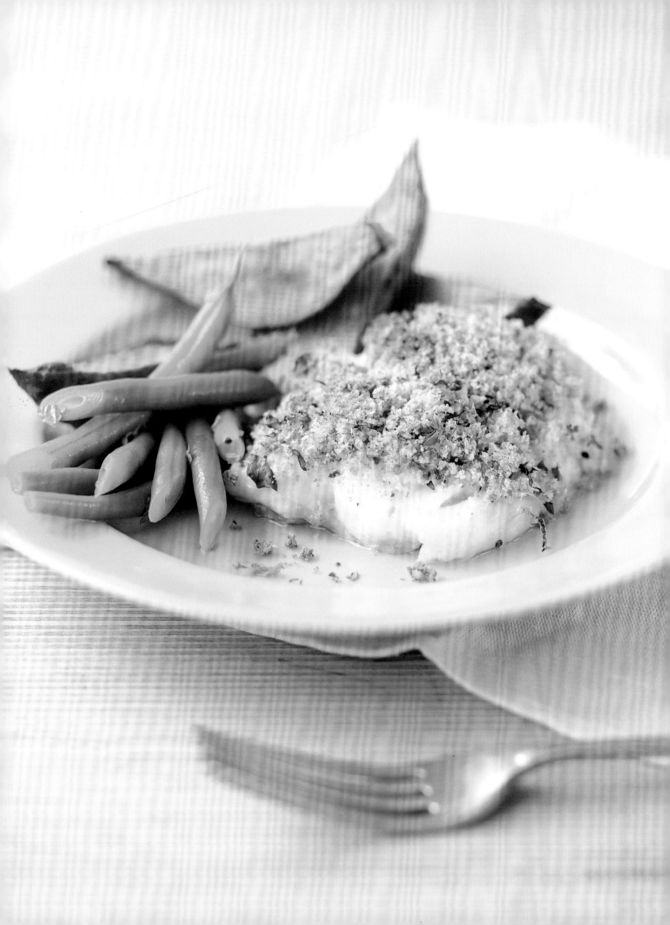

grilled teriyaki salmon

with cucumber ribbons & sesame rice

sweet and aromatic teriyaki salmon makes a tempting dinner for family and friends.

Ingredients

2.5-cm (1-in) piece ginger, peeled and grated

2 tbsp low-salt soy sauce

2 tbsp rice wine

4 tsp runny honey

3 tsp sesame oil

4 skinless salmon fillets, about 120 g (4 oz) each

4 tbsp rice or white wine vinegar

20-cm (8-in) piece cucumber, peeled into 'ribbons' with a vegetable peeler

4 tsp toasted sesame seeds

240 g (8½ oz) long-grain brown rice

1 lime, cut into wedges

coriander leaves, small bunch, roughly chopped

Method

1 Stir together all but 1 teaspoon of the ginger, the soy sauce, rice wine, 2 teaspoons of the honey and 1 teaspoon of the sesame oil.

2 Place the salmon fillets in a bowl and pour over the marinade, making sure that they are completely covered. Set aside for 15–20 minutes.

3 Preheat the grill to medium–high. Rinse the brown rice well and cook according to packet instructions. Meanwhile, stir together the remaining honey with the rice wine vinegar and pour over the cucumber ribbons. Set aside.

4 Grill the salmon for 5–8 minutes, until just cooked through, pouring over any excess marinade as you go.

5 Stir the remaining oil and the sesame seeds into the rice and serve the salmon on a bed of rice with the cucumber ribbons and a wedge of lime on the side. Scatter with coriander leaves.

Tips & variations

For a vegetarian alternative use 1 packet of firm tofu, approximately 400 g (14 oz), sliced into 4. Marinate in the same way and grill for 2 minutes on each side (represents 2 protein servings).

SERVINGS		NUTRITION	
2½	Carbohydrates	524	Calories
4	Protein	61 g	Carbohydrates
½	Fat	30 g	Protein
0	Dairy	4 g	Fibre
1	Vegetables	0.5 g	Salt
0	Fruit		

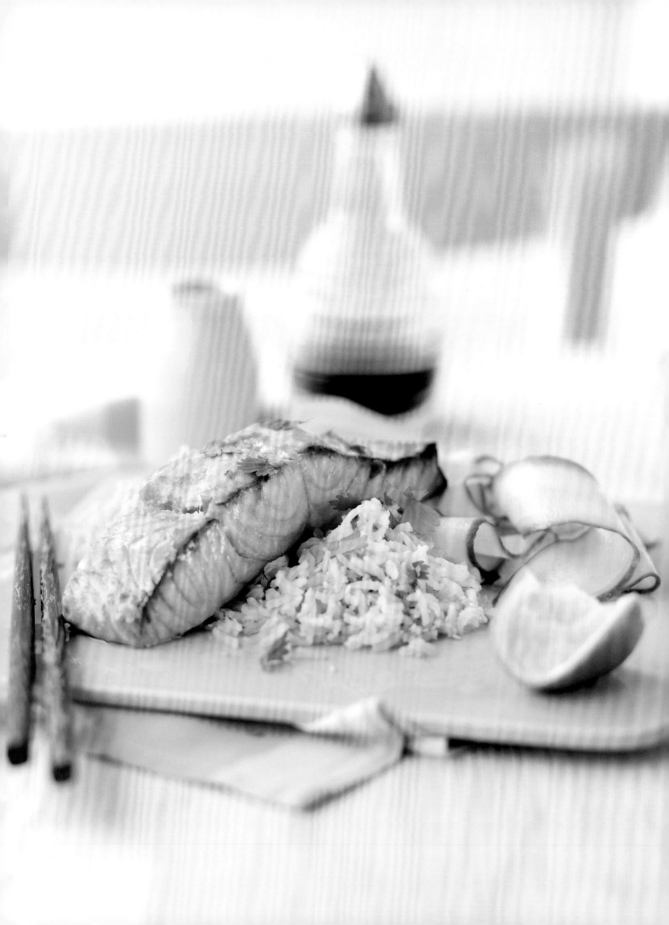

fish pie with a celeriac & potato rosti topping

A wholesome and comforting family dinner.

Ingredients

360 g (12½ oz) floury potatoes, peeled and halved if large

360 g (12½ oz) celeriac, peeled and cut into large chunks (about the same size as the potatoes)

120 g (4 oz) low-fat herby cream cheese

150 ml (5 fl oz/¼ pint) low-salt fish or vegetable stock

2 tbsp arrowroot, mixed with 2 tbsp water

1 tbsp Dijon mustard

8 spring onions, finely sliced

240 g (8½ oz) undyed smoked haddock, cut into bite-sized pieces

240 g (8½ oz) salmon fillets, cut into bite-sized pieces

180 g (6⅓ oz) raw tiger prawns, thawed if frozen and patted dry

4 eggs, boiled for 7 minutes, peeled and sliced

100 g (3½ oz) baby spinach leaves

1 tbsp parsley, chopped

2 tsp olive oil

black pepper

Method

1 Begin by making the rosti topping. Place the potatoes and celeriac in a pan of boiling water and simmer for 10 minutes. Drain and set aside to cool.

2 Preheat the oven to 190°C/375°F/gas mark 5. Now make the sauce. Melt the cream cheese in a saucepan over a medium–low heat. Gradually stir in the stock until smooth, followed by the arrowroot. Bring up to a boil and simmer, stirring, for 2 minutes, until thickened.

3 Remove from the heat and stir in the mustard and half the spring onions. Arrange the fish, prawns, egg slices and spinach leaves in an ovenproof dish, about 1.5 litres (2½ pints) in capacity. Sprinkle over half the parsley and season well with black pepper. Pour over the sauce, making sure to cover all the filling.

4 Now grate the potato and celeriac, mix with the remaining spring onions and parsley and the oil. Season with pepper and spoon over the fish pie filling evenly.

5 Bake for 30 minutes, until the sauce is bubbling and the pie is piping hot.

Tips & variations

Instead of grating the celeriac and potato, you can mash it after boiling. Stir through the remaining spring onions and the parsley, season with black pepper before spooning over the pie filling and baking as per the recipe.

SERVINGS		NUTRITION	
1½	Carbohydrates	497	Calories
5	Protein	34 g	Carbohydrates
0	Fat	46 g	Protein
1	Dairy	5 g	Fibre
1½	Vegetables	2.3 g	Salt
0	Fruit		

harissa pork burgers

with cinnamon, squash wedges & minted yoghurt

The flavour of pork is perfectly enhanced by spicy harissa and cinnamon-roasted squash.

Ingredients

480 g (1 lb 1 oz) lean pork mince

1 tbsp harissa

4 spring onions, finely sliced

1 slice wholemeal bread, whizzed into breadcrumbs

1 tbsp flat-leaf parsley, finely chopped

1 egg, beaten

320 g (11 oz) butternut squash, peeled and cut into wedges (no need to peel)

1 tsp ground cinnamon

2 tsp olive oil

150 g (5 oz) low-fat Greek yoghurt

2 tbsp mint leaves, finely chopped

160 g (5½ oz) salad leaves

1 lemon, cut into wedges

black pepper

Method

1 Place the pork mince in a mixing bowl and mix with the harissa, spring onions, breadcrumbs and parsley. Stir in enough egg to bring the mince together – you may not need to use all of it.

2 Season well with black pepper and divide the mince into 8, forming into patties. Refrigerate the patties for 30 minutes.

3 Preheat the oven to 200°C/400°F/gas mark 6. Toss the butternut squash in the cinnamon and oil and season with black pepper. Tumble the squash on to a baking tray and roast for 20–25 minutes, turning halfway through, until golden and sticky.

4 Meanwhile, preheat the grill to medium–high. Remove the pork burgers from the fridge 10 minutes before cooking. Grill the burgers for 4–5 minutes on each side, until golden brown and piping hot right through.

5 Stir together the yoghurt and mint. Serve the burgers with the wedges, dolloped with the yoghurt and with the salad leaves and a wedge of lemon on the side.

Tips & variations

You can also use ordinary plain yoghurt (whole-milk or low-fat) or low-fat fromage frais instead of low-fat Greek yoghurt.

SERVINGS		NUTRITION	
0	Carbohydrates	295	Calories
4	Protein	14 g	Carbohydrates
0	Fat	29 g	Protein
0	Dairy	3 g	Fibre
1½	Vegetables	0.5 g	Salt
0	Fruit		

mustard pork & apples

with crisp potatoes & green beans

This beautifully simple dish is a great alternative to a Sunday roast.

Ingredients

small, floury potatoes, about 120 g (4 oz) each, peeled and very finely sliced

3 tsp olive oil

480 g (1 lb 1 oz) pork fillet, trimmed of fat and sinew and cut into rounds about 2-cm (¾-in) thick (allow 2–3 slices per person)

2 sharp eating apples, such as Braeburn or Cox's, cored and cut into wedges

250 ml (9 fl oz) low-salt chicken stock

1 tbsp wholegrain mustard

1 tbsp sage leaves, roughly chopped

1 tsp thyme leaves, chopped

320 g (11 oz) green beans

black pepper

Method

1 Preheat the oven to 200°C/400°F/gas mark 6. Toss the potato slices in 2 teaspoons of the oil, season with black pepper and transfer to a baking tray, making sure that the potatoes do not overlap too much. Bake for 20 minutes or so, until the potatoes are golden brown at the edges and quite crisp.

2 Meanwhile, heat the remaining oil in a large frying pan over a medium–high heat. Fry the pork for 2–3 minutes on each side, until nicely browned. Remove from the pan and tip the apple wedges into the pan. Fry for 2–3 minutes, turning every so often, until golden.

3 Return the pork to the pan, add the stock and simmer for a further 2–3 minutes, until the pork is cooked through. Stir in the mustard and herbs and season with black pepper. Remove from the heat. Meanwhile blanch the beans in boiling water for 2 minutes and drain.

4 Serve the pork and apples with the sauce, and the crisp potatoes and beans on the side.

SERVINGS		NUTRITION	
1	Carbohydrates	326	Calories
4	Protein	30 g	Carbohydrates
0	Fat	32 g	Protein
0	Dairy	6 g	Fibre
1	Vegetables	0.5 g	Salt
½	Fruit		

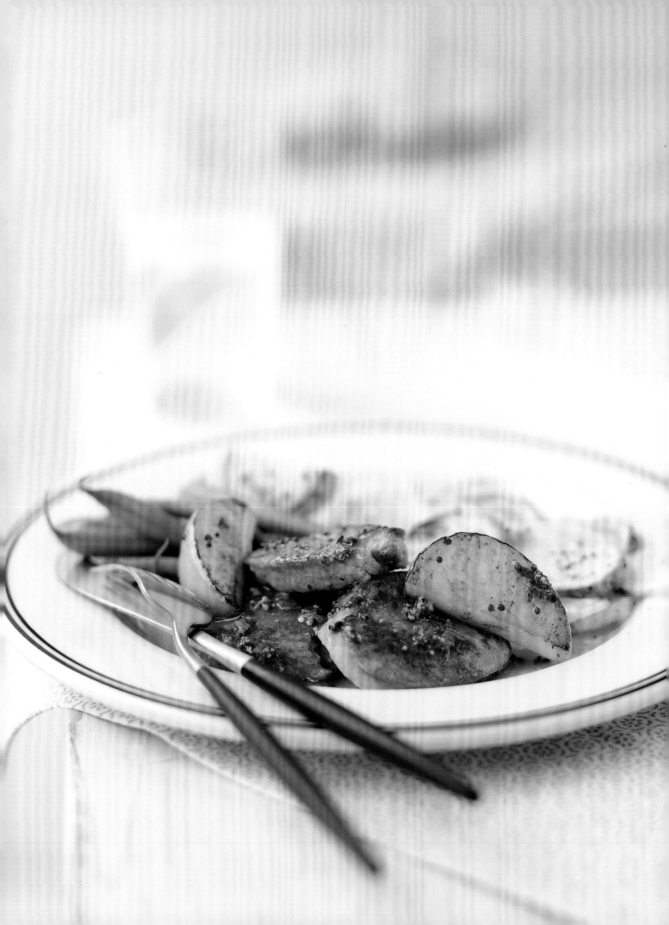

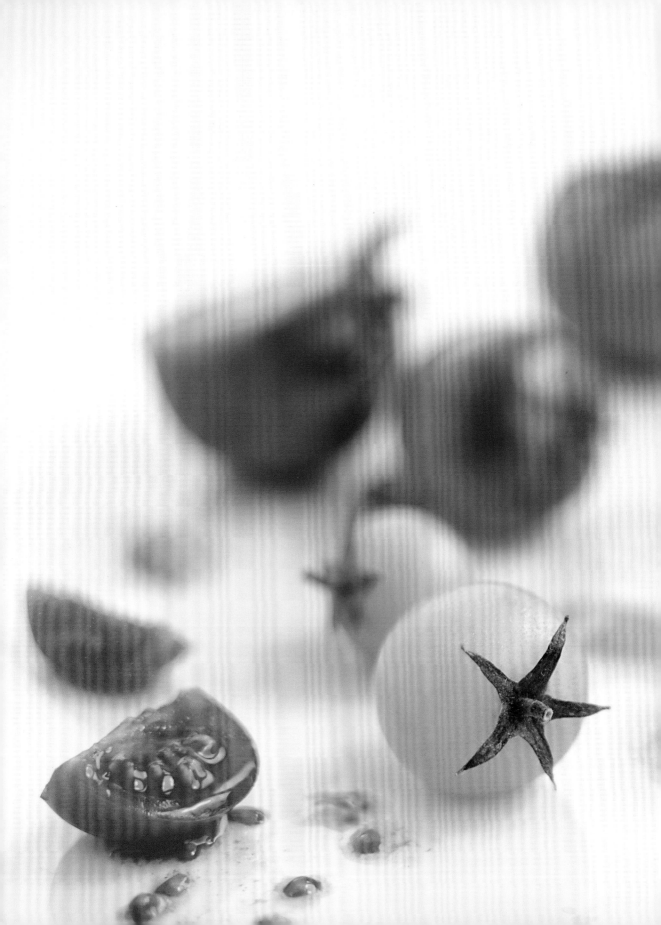

unrestricted days
classic vegetarian mains

lemon-scented quinoa & spring vegetable risotto

Starchy risotto rice is replaced with light and nutritious quinoa to make a zingy risotto.

Ingredients

2 tsp olive oil

1 onion, finely chopped

2 cloves garlic, crushed

240 g (8½ oz) quinoa

900 ml (1½ pints) hot, low-salt vegetable stock

160 g (5½ oz) broccoli, cut into small florets

160 g (5½ oz) asparagus, trimmed and cut into 2.5-cm (1-in) pieces

240 g (8½ oz) soya beans, thawed if frozen

1 lemon, zest

1 tbsp thyme leaves, roughly chopped

30 g (1 oz) Parmesan, grated

black pepper

Method

1 Heat the oil in a large frying pan over a medium heat. Add the onion and cook gently for 5 minutes, until it has softened but not browned.

2 Add the garlic and cook for 1 minute, until fragrant. Stir in the quinoa and cook, stirring, for 1–2 minutes. Pour in enough stock to cover the quinoa grains, turn the heat down to a simmer and stir until the stock has almost been absorbed.

3 Continue to add the stock in this way, until there is about one-fifth left and the quinoa has been cooking for about 9 minutes.

4 Add the vegetables and the remaining stock and cook for a further 3 minutes, or until the quinoa has softened and most of the liquid has been absorbed.

5 Remove from the heat, season well with black pepper and stir through the lemon zest, thyme and Parmesan. Serve immediately.

Tips & variations

Risotto should be loose in texture. When adding the last of the stock, allow most to be absorbed, but serve before the quinoa dries out.

SERVINGS		NUTRITION	
1	Carbohydrates	334	Calories
1	Protein	42 g	Carbohydrates
0	Fat	21 g	Protein
0	Dairy	6 g	Fibre
1½	Vegetables	1 g	Salt
0	Fruit		

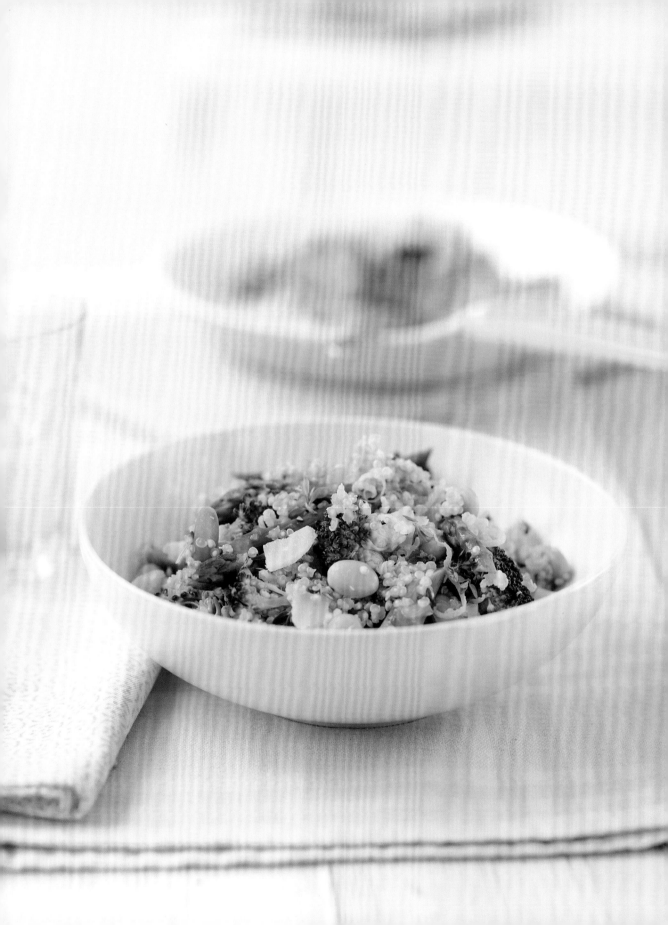

vegetarian cottage pie

with a butternut squash & sweet potato topping

Traditional veggie cottage pie is given a twist by adding rich porcini mushrooms.

Ingredients

4 tsp olive oil

1 medium onion, chopped

2 medium carrots, peeled and roughly chopped

2 sticks celery, finely chopped

350 g (12 oz) packet Quorn mince

2 tbsp tomato purée

1 tbsp vegetarian Worcester sauce or soy sauce

4 tbsp dried and finely sliced porcini mushrooms, soaked in 120 ml (4 fl oz) boiling water for 10 minutes

1 tbsp thyme leaves, roughly chopped

350 ml (12 fl oz) vegetable stock

2 small sweet potatoes (about 90 g/3 oz each), peeled and cut into 0.5-cm (¼-in) thick slices

160 g (5½ oz) butternut squash, peeled and sliced into 0.5-cm (¼-in) thick slices

black pepper

Method

1 Preheat the oven to 200°C/400°F/gas mark 6. Heat the oil in a large saucepan or casserole over a medium heat. Add the onion, carrots and celery and cook, stirring occasionally, for 5–8 minutes, until softened.

2 Add the Quorn mince, tomato purée and Worcester sauce, followed by the mushrooms, along with 4 tablespoons of the soaking liquor, the thyme and the vegetable stock. Bring everything up to a simmer and cook for 10 minutes, stirring occasionally, until slightly reduced.

3 Meanwhile, blanch the sweet potato and butternut squash in boiling water for 3–4 minutes and drain well.

4 Season the pie filling with black pepper and transfer to a pie dish. Layer up the potato and squash slices to cover the pie filling and drizzle over any remaining oil. Bake in the oven for 30 minutes, until the filling is bubbling and the top is golden brown.

Tips & variations

This dish can be made ahead of time and frozen before the stage at which it goes into the oven. You can use 150 g (5 oz) of dried TVP instead of Quorn, if preferred. Rehydrate according to packet instructions and use in the same way. Substitute the dried porcini for fresh mushrooms if preferred.

SERVINGS		NUTRITION	
½	Carbohydrates	205	Calories
3	Protein	22 g	Carbohydrates
½	Fat	16 g	Protein
0	Dairy	11 g	Fibre
2	Vegetables	1.5 g	Salt
0	Fruit		

twice-baked cheese & leek potato soufflés

These baked potatoes are a great comfort food.

Ingredients

4 baking potatoes, about 120 g (4 oz) each, scrubbed and dried

3 tsp olive oil

2 medium leeks, finely sliced

2 tsp thyme leaves, roughly chopped

2 eggs, separated

2 tsp wholegrain mustard

60 g (2 oz) low-fat Cheddar or Edam, grated

160 g (5½ oz) salad leaves

black pepper

Tips & variations

You can bake the potatoes the day before, leave them to cool and refrigerate overnight – before the cutting and mashing stage.

Method

1 Preheat the oven to 200°C/400°F/gas mark 6. Rub the potatoes all over with 1 teaspoon of the oil and place on a baking tray. Bake in the oven for 45 minutes to 1 hour, until the potatoes are tender and the skin is crisp. Remove from the oven and set aside to cool slightly.

2 Meanwhile, place a frying pan over a low–medium heat and add the remaining oil. Add the leeks to the pan and cook gently, stirring occasionally, until soft and slightly golden at the edges – this should take about 10 minutes. Add the thyme and set aside.

3 When the potatoes are cool enough to handle, cut each in half and scoop out most of the flesh into a mixing bowl. Mash the flesh until light and fluffy before stirring in the leek and thyme mixture. If hot, leave to cool for a few minutes. Stir in the egg yolks, wholegrain mustard and cheese, until completely combined. Season with black pepper.

4 In a separate bowl, whisk the egg whites until they form medium–stiff peaks. Carefully fold the egg white into the potato mix, being careful not to knock out too much air. Spoon the potato mix back into the skins and return to the oven for 10–15 minutes, until the filling has puffed up and is golden. Serve immediately with the salad leaves.

SERVINGS		NUTRITION	
1	Carbohydrates	220	Calories
½	Protein	23 g	Carbohydrates
0	Fat	13 g	Protein
½	Dairy	5 g	Fibre
1½	Vegetables	0.5 g	Salt
0	Fruit		

bean & cheese quesadillas

When you're in a hurry, Mexican quesadillas make a great store-cupboard dinner.

Ingredients

4 tsp olive oil

2 small onions, finely chopped

4 cloves garlic, crushed

1 tsp chilli powder

½ tsp ground cumin

1 tsp smoked sweet paprika

2 x 400 g (14 oz) tins kidney beans, rinsed and drained

8 medium tomatoes, chopped

4 large seeded tortilla wraps

120 g (4 oz) low-fat Cheddar or Edam, grated

8 spring onions, finely sliced

coriander leaves, large handful, roughly chopped

320 g (11 oz) salad leaves

2 limes, cut into wedges

Method

1 Heat the oil in a large frying pan over a medium heat. Add the onion and cook gently for 5–8 minutes, until softened. Add the garlic, chilli powder, cumin and paprika and cook, stirring, for 1 minute, until fragrant. Add the beans and tomatoes and cook for 2–3 minutes, until heated through.

2 Heat a frying pan large enough to hold the tortillas over a medium heat, then add one of the tortillas. Spoon half of the bean mixture across the tortilla, leaving a 1-cm (½-inch) border around the edge. Sprinkle with half the cheese and spring onion and top with another tortilla, pressing down lightly to hold them together.

3 Dry-fry for a further minute then carefully slide the quesadilla onto a large plate. Put another large plate on top, invert it, then slide the quesadilla back into the frying pan to cook for 2 minutes on the other side, until golden brown, cheese melted. Repeat with the remaining tortillas.

4 Cut each quesadilla in half and serve scattered with coriander, salad leaves and lime wedges on the side.

Tips & variations

If you don't have a frying pan large enough to fit the tortillas, bake them on an baking tray at 200°C/400°F/gas mark 6 for 8–10 minutes, until the cheese has melted.

SERVINGS		NUTRITION	
2	Carbohydrates	472	Calories
2	Protein	66 g	Carbohydrates
½	Fat	26 g	Protein
1	Dairy	14 g	Fibre
3½	Vegetables	2.5 g	Salt
0	Fruit		

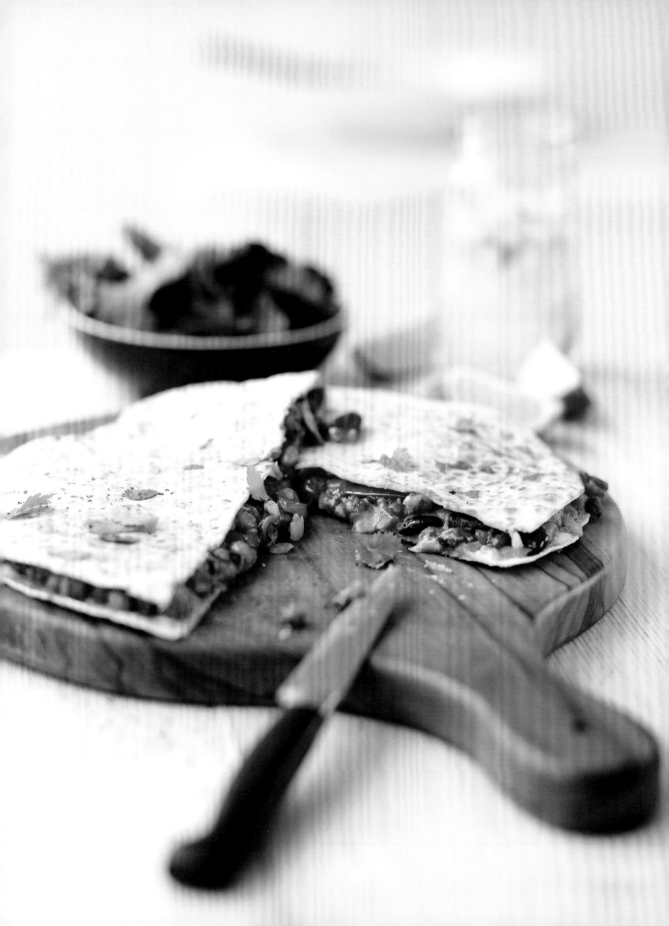

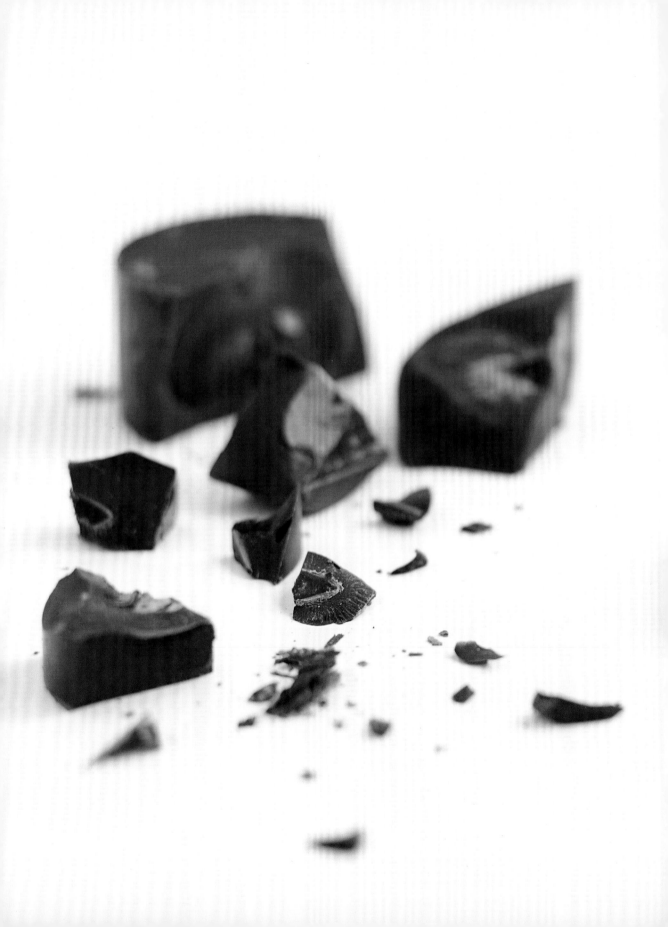

unrestricted days
desserts & baking

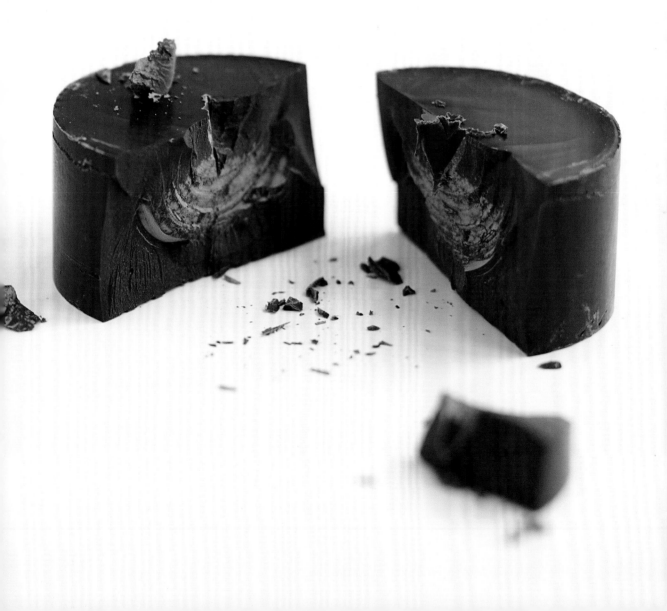

banana & chocolate loaf cake

This moist cake is a perfect guilt-free tea-time treat.

Ingredients

a little oil, for greasing

150 g (5 oz) wholemeal self-raising flour

¾ tsp baking powder

250 g (9 oz) very ripe bananas, mashed

2 tbsp runny honey

2 large eggs, beaten

100 g (3½ oz) low-fat natural yoghurt

35 g (1¼ oz) toasted hazelnuts, roughly chopped

40 g (1⅓ oz) dark chocolate (at least 70 per cent cocoa solids), roughly chopped

Method

1 Preheat the oven to 160°C/325°F/gas mark 3. Lightly grease a 1.5-litre (2½-pint) loaf tin and fully line with baking parchment.

2 Sift the flour and baking powder into a large mixing bowl and make a well in the centre. In a separate bowl, mix together the bananas, honey, eggs, yoghurt and half the hazelnuts and chocolate. Pour the wet mixture into the dry and quickly and lightly fold together to make a batter. Stop mixing as soon as all the ingredients are combined and scrape the mixture into the lined tin.

3 Bake for 1 to 1 hour 15 minutes, until golden brown and a skewer inserted into the middle comes out clean. Allow to cool slightly on a wire rack. Melt the remaining chocolate gently in the microwave for 40 seconds to 1 minute or in a bowl over a saucepan of hot water. Drizzle the melted chocolate over the cake and scatter with the remaining hazelnuts. Allow to set slightly before serving.

Tips & variations

Really ripe bananas will make for a rich, sweet cake.

SERVINGS		NUTRITION	
1	Carbohydrates	199	Calories
0	Protein	31 g	Carbohydrates
½	Fat	6 g	Protein
0	Dairy	3 g	Fibre
0	Vegetables	0.3 g	Salt
½	Fruit		

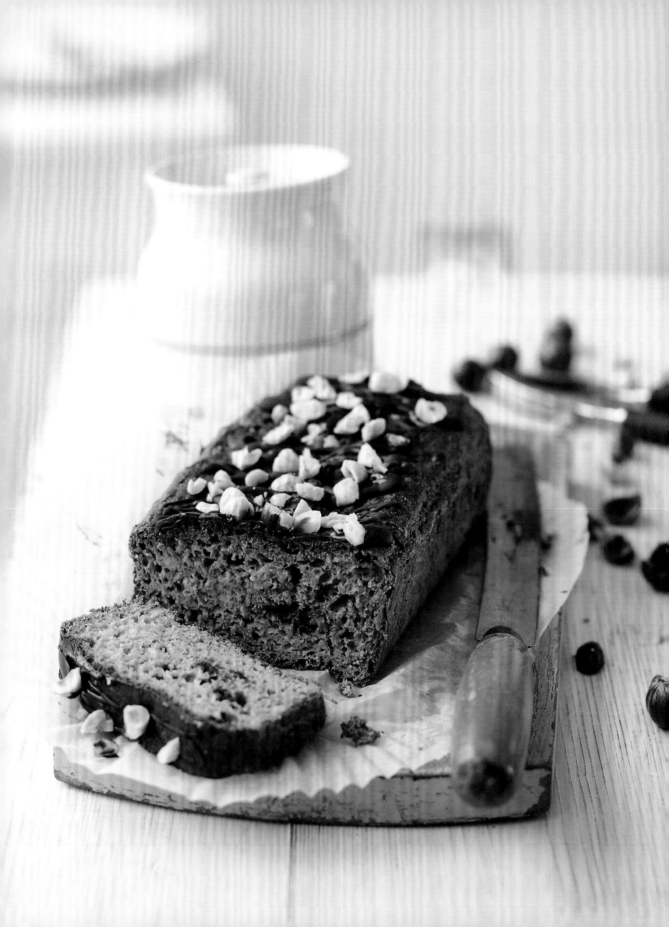

mini banoffee pies

Traditionally calorific, banoffee pies are lightened with creamy Greek yoghurt.

Ingredients

100 g (3½ oz) Grape Nuts, whizzed quickly in a food processor to make crumbs

½ orange, juice and zest

20 g (¾ oz) Demerara sugar

4 tsp low-fat spread, melted

2 small bananas, sliced

4 tsp runny honey

200 g (7 oz) low-fat Greek yoghurt

20 g (¾ oz) dark chocolate (at least 70 per cent cocoa solids), grated

Method

1 Stir together the Grape Nut crumbs, orange juice and zest, sugar and melted low-fat spread. Divide between 4 small bowls or tumbler glasses, sprinkling rather than pressing the mixture. Refrigerate for 10 minutes to firm up.

2 Lay the banana slices over the crumb mixture in concentric circles and drizzle over the honey.

3 Spoon over the Greek yoghurt and finish by scattering with grated chocolate. The 'pies' can be served straightaway or refrigerated for up to 2 hours before serving.

Tips & variations

Grape Nuts are high in fibre and can be found with the breakfast cereals in most supermarkets.

SERVINGS		NUTRITION	
2	Carbohydrates	290	Calories
0	Protein	51 g	Carbohydrates
1	Fat	6 g	Protein
½	Dairy	3 g	Fibre
0	Vegetables	0.6 g	Salt
½	Fruit		
1	Treat		

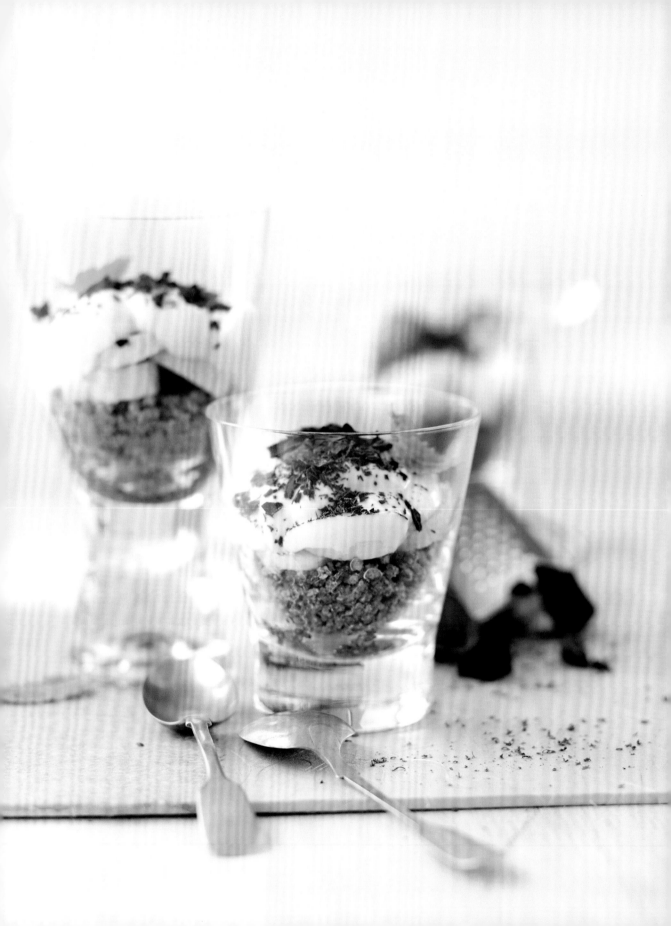

hot-cross bun & butter pudding

This twist on the classic bread and butter pudding is delicately spiced and a delicious sweet treat.

Ingredients

4 fruit hot-cross buns, cut in half horizontally

4 tsp low-fat spread

6 semi-dried figs, finely chopped

2 eggs, lightly beaten

400 ml (13 fl oz) semi-skimmed milk

30 g (1 oz) Demerara sugar

¼ tsp ground cinnamon

½ orange, zest

Method

1 Heat the oven to 170°C/338°F/gas mark 3. Spread the buns with the low-fat spread and place in an ovenproof dish, about 1.5 litres (2½ pints) in capacity. Sprinkle over the figs.

2 Beat together the eggs, milk, sugar, cinnamon and orange zest and pour over the bun halves, making sure that they are entirely covered. Leave to soak for 15 minutes before baking in the oven for 40–45 minutes, until golden brown and just set. Serve immediately.

Tips & variations

If you aren't a fan of cinnamon, use a few grates of fresh nutmeg, the bashed seeds of 2 cardamom pods or the seeds of half a vanilla pod instead.

SERVINGS		NUTRITION	
2½	Carbohydrates	398	Calories
½	Protein	61 g	Carbohydrates
1	Fat	12 g	Protein
½	Dairy	6 g	Fibre
0	Vegetables	0.6 g	Salt
1	Fruit		
1	Treat		

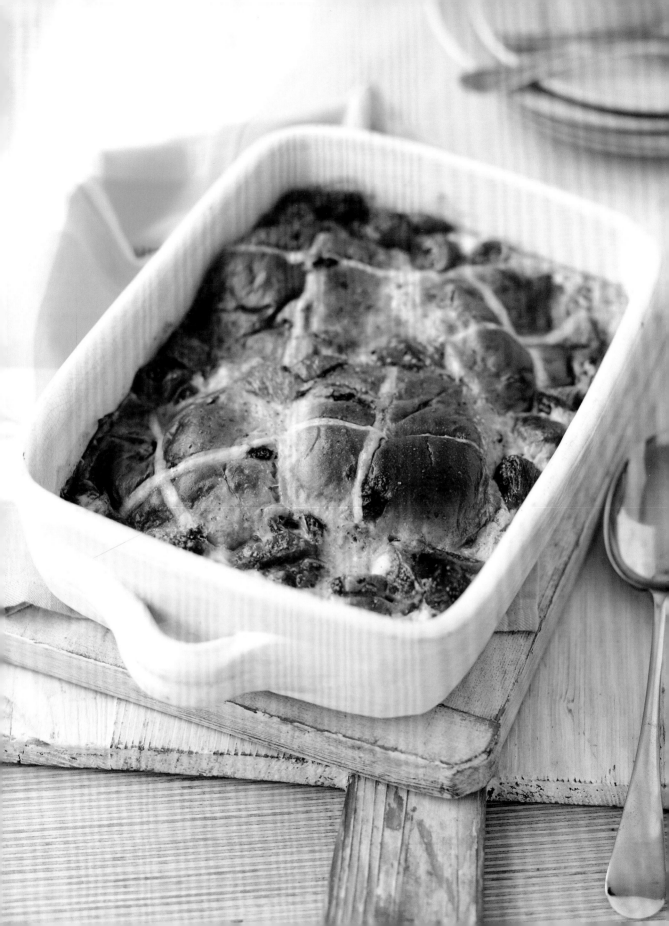

fruit & hazelnut soda bread

This rich, fruity loaf is ideal for the amateur bread-maker to try.

Ingredients

200 g (7 oz) wholemeal flour

100 g (3½ oz) plain flour

15 g (½ oz) low-fat spread

75 g (2½ oz) jumbo porridge oats

1 tsp bicarbonate of soda

20 g (¾ oz) caster sugar

75 g (2½ oz) mixed dried fruit, such as currants, raisins and cranberries

50 g (1¾ oz) toasted hazelnuts, roughly chopped

300 ml (10 fl oz/½ pint) buttermilk or 300 g (10½ oz) low-fat hazelnut yoghurt

Method

1 Preheat the oven to 200°C/400°F/gas mark 6. Sift both types of flour into a bowl and, using your fingertips, rub the spread into the flour. Add the porridge oats, bicarbonate of soda, caster sugar, dried fruit and hazelnuts and stir well to combine.

2 Pour the buttermilk or yoghurt into the middle of the dry mix and quickly and lightly bring the mixture together. Stop mixing as soon as it forms a dough. Form the mixture into a ball and transfer to a lightly floured baking tray. Press the top of the bread down to flatten slightly and, using the handle of a wooden spoon, create a cross shape deep into the bread.

3 Bake for 30–35 minutes, until the bread is golden and the bread sounds hollow when the underside is tapped.

4 Allow to cool, covered with a tea towel, on a wire rack before slicing.

Tips & variations

The soda bread can be frozen once cooled completely. Defrost at room temperature and warm in the oven before serving with low-fat spread or light cream cheese.

SERVINGS		NUTRITION	
3	Carbohydrates	345	Calories
0	Protein	59 g	Carbohydrates
1	Fat	10 g	Protein
1	Dairy	7 g	Fibre
0	Vegetables	0.1 g	Salt
½	Fruit		

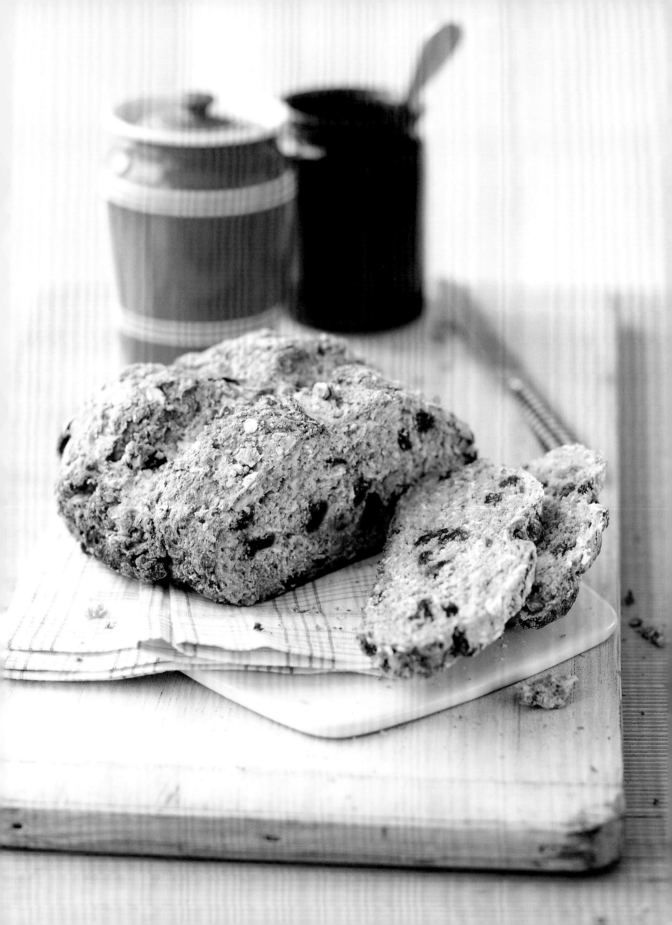

recipes summary

Use this chart as a quick reference to the nutritional information and servings for each recipe in the book. **V** indicates that the recipe is suitable for vegetarians; **VT** indicates vegetarian tip – that the recipe includes advice on adapting it for vegetarians.

| RESTRICTED DAYS RECIPES | PAGE | SERVINGS PER RECIPE |||||| NUTRITIONAL INFORMATION IN GRAMS |||||
		CARBS	PROTEIN	FAT	DAIRY	VEG	FRUIT	CALORIES	CARBS	PROTEIN	FIBRE	SALT
Breakfasts	14											
Boiled eggs/asparagus/ham VT	16	0	3	0	0	1	0	231	2	23	2	1.3
Skinny English breakfast VT	18	0	3	½	0	2	0	282	5	26	2	3.2
Spiced tofu scramble V	19	0	2	0	0	1	0	111	2	10	3	0.2
Grilled kipper/poached egg VT	20	0	4	0	0	1	0	261	3	22	2	1.6
Raspberry & strawberry smoothie V	22	0	0	0	1½	0	1	148	18	11	4	0.4
Soups	24											
Spring green V	26	0	1½	0	½	1½	0	150	6	14	6	1.1
Spiced pumpkin, tomato & spinach V	28	0	0	0	0	2	0	52	6	3	3	1.1
Indonesian chicken	29	0	2½	0	0	½	0	143	3	19	1	1.1
Saffron fish	30	0	2	0	0	1½	0	116	4	20	3	1.2
Salads & packed lunches	32											
Spring fennel V	34	0	2	½	0	2½	0	135	6	10	8	<0.1
Halloumi, watermelon & mint V	36	0	0	1	2	½	1	224	7	10	2	2.3
Tofu & mushroom spring rolls V	38	0	2	½	0	1½	0	116	2	11	3	0.2
Smoked mackerel VT	39	0	4	½	0	1	0	471	3	28	2	2.3
Crab, melon & rocket VT	40	0	2	½	0	½	1	173	5	20	2	1.1
Bang bang chicken VT	42	0	4	1	0	2½	0	219	6	31	3	2
Green bean, broccoli & chicken	44	0	4	1	0	3	0	245	7	34	7	0.3
Pesto turkey	45	0	4	1	0	2½	0	209	7	32	3	0.5
30-minute meals	46											
Piri piri turkey & pepper skewers VT	48	0	2	0	0	2½	0	107	7	18	3	0.3
Open spiced turkey burgers	50	0	4	1	0	½	0	255	2	32	3	1
Grilled miso chicken VT	52	0	4	0	0	2	0	189	5	30	3	0.9
Stuffed tarragon chicken	54	0	5	0	1	1	0	278	3	39	1	1.7
Chicken & spinach curry VT	56	0	4	0	½	1½	0	242	12	35	4	0.6
Asian duck, grapefruit & watercress	57	0	4	0	0	1	1	229	8	27	2.5	0.7
Griddled tuna steak	58	0	4	0	0	2	1	255	12	31	5	0.2
Lemon & garlic prawns	60	0	4	½	0	½	0	197	5	26	5	0.6
Herb-stuffed trout	61	8	4	0	0	1½	½	210	8	26	4	2
Mustard salmon	62	6	4	0	0	2½	0	290	6	29	5	0.5
Baked smoked haddock VT	63	2	3½	0	0	1	0	252	2	39	2	3.4
Goan spiced mackerel	64	9	4	0	½	1½	0	347	9	28	2	0.4
Chimichurri steak VT	66	4	4	½	0	1½	0	202	4	28	2	0.2
Thai beef salad VT	68	3	4	0	0	1½	0	192	3	28	2	0.3
Lamb steaks	70	4	4	0	0	2	0	249	4	29	3	0.4
Herb & mustard-crusted pork fillet	72	6	4	0	0	2½	0	217	6	30	4	0.8

RESTRICTED DAYS RECIPES

RESTRICTED DAYS RECIPES	PAGE	SERVINGS PER RECIPE						NUTRITIONAL INFORMATION IN GRAMS				
		CARBS	PROTEIN	FAT	DAIRY	VEG	FRUIT	CALORIES	CARBS	PROTEIN	FIBRE	SALT
Moroccan spiced pork fillet	74	0	4	0	0	1½	0	177	2	28	3	0.2
Venison & blackberries	75	0	4	½	0	1½	½	192	5	30	4	1.3
Quick & easy vegetarian mains	76											
Middle-Eastern kale salad V	78	0	2	0	½	1	0	277	7	23	2	0.7
Okra & tomato curry V	80	0	0	0	1½	2	0	145	10	9	5	0.3
Smoked aubergine salad V	82	0	2	0	0	3	0	146	10	11	9	<0.1
Soya bean burger V	83	0	2	3½	0	2	0	335	10	20	9	0.1
Stuffed courgettes V	84	0	0	½	1	1½	0	144	3	7	2	1.2
Desserts	86											
Instant blackberry frozen yoghurt V	88	0	0	0	½	0	1	79	10	5	4	0.2
Melon, mint & pineapple granita V	90	0	0	0	0	0	1	14	3	0	1	<0.1
Rhubarb fool V	91	0	0	½	½	0	1	88	7	6	2	0.2

UNRESTRICTED DAYS RECIPES

UNRESTRICTED DAYS RECIPES	PAGE	SERVINGS PER RECIPE						NUTRITIONAL INFORMATION IN GRAMS				
		CARBS	PROTEIN	FAT	DAIRY	VEG	FRUIT	CALORIES	CARBS	PROTEIN	FIBRE	SALT
Breakfasts	94											
Banana/flaxseed pancakes V	96	1½	0	½	0	0	½	218	37	7	5	0.1
Baked ham & eggs in bread cups VT	98	1	1½	½	½	0	0	257	16	20	3	1.8
Lunches on the go	100											
Herbed quinoa salad V	102	2	0	1	1	2½	½	430	61	16	3	1.2
Chicken noodle salad VT	104	1	4	1	0	1½	0	374	42	34	4	1.1
Hot-smoked salmon, orange, potato	106	1	2	1	0	1	0	259	24	20	5	3
Quick mackerel & horseradish pâté	107	1	1½	0	1	1	0	384	40	17	9	1.3
Favourite dinners	108											
Turkey, tarragon & mushroom pie	110	1	4	0	1	1½	0	299	20	36	5	1.1
One-pot chicken & veg	112	0	4	0	0	2½	0	221	14	30	5	0.3
Braised French chicken	113	0	4½	0	½	1½	0	239	5	35	4	1.4
Roasted cod	114	1½	3	½	0	1	0	308	30	37	6	0.6
Grilled teriyaki salmon VT	116	2½	4	½	0	1	0	524	61	30	4	0.5
Fish pie	118	1½	5	0	1	1½	0	497	34	46	5	2.3
Harissa pork burgers	119	0	4	0	0	1½	0	295	14	29	3	0.5
Mustard pork & apples	120	1	4	0	0	1	½	326	30	32	6	0.5
Classic vegetarian mains	122											
Lemon-scented quinoa V	124	1	1	0	0	1½	0	334	42	21	6	1
Vegetarian cottage pie V	126	½	3	½	0	2	0	205	22	16	11	1.5
Twice-baked cheese soufflé V	127	1	½	0	½	1½	0	220	23	13	5	0.5
Bean & cheese quesadillas V	128	2	2	½	1	3½	0	472	66	26	14	2.5
Desserts & baking	130											
Banana & chocolate loaf cake V	132	1	0	½	0	0	½	199	31	6	3	0.3
Mini banoffee pies V	134	2	0	1	½	0	½	290	51	6	3	0.6
Hot-cross bun & butter pudding V	136	2½	½	1	½	0	1	398	61	12	6	0.6
Fruit & hazelnut soda bread V	138	3	0	1	1	½	½	345	59	10	7	0.1

serving sizes for the two restricted days

The Ready Reckoners on pages 146–9 explain how many servings of each food you should eat. The food lists below show serving sizes for the many different foods allowed on restricted days. Try to eat the minimum protein and all of your vegetable, dairy and fruit allowance. Vegetarians can choose four servings from the dairy list, two of which should be lower-fat cheeses, and are allowed more vegetable proteins from the list below.

Weights are given for raw meat and fish. Cooked meats will weigh about one-third less than raw, with one serving equivalent to 20 g cooked meat, poultry and oily fish and 40 g of white fish.

CARBOHYDRATE FOODS	SERVINGS
Carbohydrate foods are not allowed on the two restricted days of the 2-Day Diet.	0

PROTEIN FOODS/minimum 4 servings per day	1 SERVING EQUAL TO:
Fresh or smoked* white fish (e.g. haddock or cod)	60 g (2 oz) (2 fish-finger-sized pieces)
Seafood (e.g. prawns, mussels, crab)	45 g (1½ oz)
Tinned tuna in brine or spring water	45 g (1½ oz)
Oily fish (fresh or tinned) in tomato sauce or oil (drained) (e.g. mackerel, sardines, salmon, trout, tuna, smoked salmon*, smoked trout* or kippers*)	30 g (1 oz)
Chicken, turkey, duck, pheasant (cooked without skin)	30 g (1 oz) (slice the size of a playing card)
Lean beef, pork, lamb, rabbit, venison or offal (fat removed)	30 g (1 oz) (slice the size of a playing card)
Lean bacon*	1 grilled rasher
Lean ham*	2 medium slices or 4 wafer-thin slices
Eggs	1 medium/large
Tofu	50 g (1¾ oz)

VEGETABLE PROTEIN	MAXIMUM	SERVINGS
Include only one of the following foods on each restricted day. They count towards your daily protein allowance. Vegetarians can include up to 6 vegetable protein servings, but make sure you have no more than 15 g of carbohydrates per day from this list.		
Textured vegetable protein (TVP)	30 g (1 oz)	3
Soya and edamame beans	60 g (2 oz)	2
Low-fat hummus	1 tablespoon (15 g/½ oz)	1
Quorn mince, pieces, fillet	115 g (4 oz)	4
Vegetarian sausage	1 sausage	2

FAT	1 SERVING EQUAL TO:
Margarine or low-fat spread (avoid the 'buttery' types)	1 teaspoon (8 g)
Olive oil or other oil (not palm, coconut or ghee)	1 dessertspoon (7 g)
Oil-based dressing	1 dessertspoon (7 g)
Unsalted, salted*, dry-roasted* nuts (not honey-roasted), seeds (linseed/ sesame)	1 dessertspoon per serving or 3 walnut halves, 3 Brazil nuts, 4 almonds, 8 peanuts, 10 cashews or 10 pistachios (not chestnuts)
Pesto	1 teaspoon (8 g)
Mayonnaise	1 teaspoon (5 g)
Low-fat mayonnaise	1 tablespoon (15 g)
Olives*	10
Peanut butter (without palm oil)	1 teaspoon (8 g)
Cocoa powder	2 heaped tablespoons (12 g)

FAT	MAXIMUM PER DAY	SERVINGS
You can only have one of the following fatty foods on each restricted day as they contain some carbohydrate. They count towards your fat serving allowance.		
Avocado	½ pear	2
Guacamole	2 tablespoons	2
Low-fat guacamole	2 tablespoons	1

DAIRY (3 SERVINGS PER DAY)	1 SERVING EQUAL TO:
Milk (semi-skimmed or skimmed)	200 ml (⅓ pint/7 fl oz)
Soya milk (sweetened or unsweetened with added calcium)	200 ml (⅓ pint/7 fl oz)
Yoghurt: diet fruit, plain soya, Greek, natural or fromage frais (all low-fat)	1 small pot 120–150 g (4–5 oz) or 3 heaped tablespoons

DAIRY (CONTINUED)	1 SERVING EQUAL TO:
Whole-milk natural yoghurt	80–90 g (2½–3 oz) or 2 heaped tablespoons
Cottage cheese	75 g (2 ½ oz) or 2 tablespoons
Quark	⅓ pot or 3 tablespoons (90 g/3 oz)
Cream cheese (low-fat or extra-light)	1 tablespoon (30 g/1 oz)
Lower-fat cheeses: low-fat Cheddar, Edam, Bavarian smoked, feta*, Camembert, ricotta, mozzarella, low-fat halloumi, paneer made from semi-skimmed milk	Matchbox size: 30 g (1 oz) to a maximum of 120 g (4 oz) for women per week and 150 g (5 oz) for men on restricted and non-restricted days

VEGETABLES (5 SERVINGS PER DAY)	1 SERVING EQUAL TO 80 g (2½ oz)
Artichoke	2 globe hearts
Asparagus, tinned	7 spears
Asparagus, fresh	5 spears
Aubergine	⅓ medium
Beans, French	4 heaped tablespoons
Beans, runner	4 heaped tablespoons
Beansprouts, fresh	2 handfuls
Broccoli	2 florets
Brussels sprouts	8
Cabbage	⅙ small cabbage or 3 heaped tablespoons of shredded leaves
Cauliflower	8 florets
Celeriac	3 heaped tablespoons
Celery	3 sticks
Chinese leaves	⅕ head
Courgette	½ large
Cucumber	5-cm (2-in) piece
Curly kale, cooked	4 heaped tablespoons
Fennel	½ cup sliced
Karela or gourd	½
Leeks	1 medium
Lettuce (mixed leaves or rocket)	1 cereal bowlful
Mangetout	1 handful
Mushrooms, fresh	14 button or 3 handfuls of sliced
Mushrooms, dried	2 tablespoons or handful porcini
Okra	16 medium
Pak choi (Chinese cabbage)	2 handfuls
Pepper (green only)	½
Pumpkin	3 heaped tablespoons
Radish	10

VEGETABLES (CONTINUED)	1 SERVING EQUAL TO 80 g (2½ oz)
Spinach, cooked	2 heaped tablespoons
Spinach, fresh	1 cereal bowlful
Spring greens, cooked	4 heaped tablespoons
Spring onion	8
Sweetcorn, baby (whole not kernels)	6
Tomato, tinned	2 plum tomatoes or ½ tin chopped
Tomato, fresh	1 medium or 7 cherry
Tomato purée	1 heaped tablespoon
Tomato, sundried	4 pieces
Watercress	1 cereal bowlful

FRUIT (1 SERVING PER DAY)	1 SERVING EQUAL TO 80 g (2½ oz)
Apricots	3 fresh or dried
Blackberries	1 handful
Blackcurrants	4 heaped tablespoons
Redcurrants	4 heaped tablespoons
Grapefruit	½ whole fruit
Melon	5-cm (2-in) slices
Pineapple	1 large slice
Papaya	1 slice
Raspberries	2 handfuls
Strawberries	7
Stewed rhubarb or cranberries, with sweetener	3 heaped tablespoons

FLAVOURINGS	SERVINGS
Lemon juice; fresh or dried herbs; spices; black pepper; mustard, horseradish, vinegars, garlic (fresh or pre-chopped); chilli (fresh or dried); soy sauce; miso paste; fish sauce; Worcester sauce	Unlimited

DRINKS	At least 8 drinks or 2 litres (4 pints) a day
Water (still or sparkling)	Unlimited
Tea and coffee, caffeinated or decaffeinated	Unlimited
Fruit, herbal or green teas	Unlimited
Sugar-free or diet squash or fizzy drinks	Up to a maximum of 9 cans (3 litres/ 6 pints) per week

* You can include 4–6 servings of these high-salt foods on each restricted day. See the box about salt on page 13.

serving sizes for the five unrestricted days

We encourage you to follow a healthy Mediterranean diet on your five unrestricted days, including carbohydrates, protein, low-fat dairy foods and a wide variety of fruits and vegetables. The tables below are a guide to what makes up a single serving of a given food. You are allowed different numbers of servings from each food group on unrestricted days, depending on your age, sex and current weight (see the Ready Reckoners, pages 146–9).

CARBOHYDRATE FOODS	1 SERVING EQUAL TO:
Wholewheat or oat breakfast cereal	3 level tablespoons (24 g/ ¾ oz), or 1 wholewheat or oat bisk
Porridge oats or sugar-free muesli	1 heaped tablespoon (20 g/²/₃ oz)
Bread: wholegrain, wholemeal, rye, granary	Medium slice, ½ roll
Pitta bread, chapatti, tortilla wrap (wholemeal or multigrain versions)	½ large
Rye crispbread	2
Wholewheat cracker	2
Wholegrain rice cake	2
Oat cake (choose a variety without palm oil)	1
Wholegrain pasta or rice	1 tablespoon uncooked (30 g/1 oz) or 2 tablespoons cooked (60 g/2 oz)
Couscous, bulgur wheat, pearl barley, quinoa	1 tablespoon uncooked (30 g/1 oz) or 2 tablespoons cooked (60 g/2 oz)
Lasagne (preferably wholemeal)	1 sheet
Noodles (preferably brown)	Half a dried block or nest (50 g/1¾ oz)
Baked or boiled potato (in skin)	1 small (120 g/4 oz) raw weight
Cassava, yam, sweet potato	1 small (90 g/3 oz) raw weight
Wholemeal pizza base	⅙ of thin medium pizza base
Sweet corn	½ corn on the cob or 2 tablespoons kernels
Wholemeal flour	Level tablespoon
Unsweetened popcorn	20 g (²/₃ oz)

PROTEIN FOODS	1 SERVING EQUAL TO:
Fresh or smoked* white fish (e.g. haddock or cod)	60 g (2 oz) (2 fish-finger-sized pieces)
Tinned tuna in brine or spring water	45 g (1½ oz)
Oily fish (fresh or tinned) in tomato sauce or oil (drained) (e. g. mackerel, sardines, salmon, trout, tuna, smoked salmon* or trout* or kippers*)	30 g (1 oz)
Seafood (e.g. prawns, mussels, crab)	45 g (1½ oz)
Chicken, pheasant, turkey or duck (cooked without skin)	30 g (1 oz) (a slice the size of a playing card)

PROTEIN FOODS (CONTINUED)	1 SERVING EQUAL TO:
Lean beef, pork, lamb, rabbit, venison or offal (fat removed)	30 g (1 oz) per serving to a maximum of 500 g (1 lb 1 oz) per week for women and 600 g (1 lb 4 oz) per week for men
Lean bacon*	1 rasher
Eggs	1 medium/large
Lean ham*	2 medium slices of 4 wafer-thin slices
Baked beans	2 level tablespoons (60 g/2 oz)
Lentils, chickpeas and beans	1 tablespoon (20 g/²/₃ oz) raw or 1½ tablespoons cooked or tinned (65 g/2 oz)
Quorn	30 g (1 oz)
Vegetarian sausage	½
Tofu	⅛ of packet (50 g/1¾ oz)
Textured vegetable protein (TVP)	1 heaped tablespoon (10 g/ ⅓ oz) uncooked
Frozen vegetarian mince	30 g (1 oz)
Low-fat hummus	1 level tablespoon (30 g/1 oz)
Soya and edamame beans	30 g (1 oz)

FAT	1 SERVING EQUAL TO:
Margarine or low-fat spread (avoid the 'buttery' types)	1 teaspoon (8 g)
Olive oil or other oil	1 dessertspoon (7 g)
Oil-based dressing	1 dessertspoon (7 g)
Unsalted nuts/seeds (e.g. sesame or linseed)	1 dessertspoon or 3 walnut halves, 3 Brazil nuts, 4 almonds, 8 peanuts, 10 cashews or pistachios
Avocado	¼ pear
Pesto	1 level teaspoon (8 g)
Olives *	10
Mayonnaise	1 teaspoon (5 g)
Guacamole or low-fat mayonnaise	1 tablespoon (15 g)
Low-fat guacamole	2 tablespoons (30 g)
Peanut butter (without palm oil)	1 heaped teaspoon (11 g)
Curry paste	1 level tablespoon (15 g)
Cocoa powder	2 heaped teaspoons (12 g)

* Try to have these salty foods only once during your five unrestricted days.

DAIRY	1 SERVING EQUAL TO:
Milk (semi-skimmed or skimmed)	200 ml (⅓ pint/7 fl oz)
Alternative 'milks' (e.g. soya, oat – sweetened or unsweetened)	200 ml (⅓ pint/7 fl oz)
Reduced-fat evaporated milk	1 level tablespoon (15 g)
Yoghurt: diet fruit, plain soya, Greek, natural or fromage frais (all low-fat)	1 small pot (120–150 g/4–5 oz) or 3 heaped tablespoons
Yoghurt: low-fat fruit, whole milk fruit and natural, flavoured soya yoghurt	80–90g (2½ – 3 oz) or 2 heaped tablespoons
Cottage cheese	¼ pot (75 g/2½ oz) or 2 tablespoons
Cream cheese (low-fat or extra-light)	1 level tablespoon (30 g/1 oz)
Quark	⅓ pot or 3 level tablespoons (90 g/3 oz)
Lower-fat cheeses: reduced-fat Cheddar, Edam, Bavarian smoked, feta*, Camembert, ricotta, mozzarella, reduced-fat halloumi, paneer made from semi-skimmed milk	Matchbox-sized: 30 g (1 oz). No more than 120 g (4 oz) per week for women and 150 g (5 oz) for men.

VEGETABLES (AT LEAST 5 PER DAY)	1 SERVING EQUAL TO 80 g (2½ oz)
Any boiled or steamed vegetables (except potato, yam, sweet corn, which are carbohydrates or pulses – counted as protein)	2–3 heaped tablespoons
Salad	1 bowl
Homemade vegetable soup	½ bowl
Vegetable juice Δ	200 ml (⅓ pint/7 fl oz)
Tomato purée	1 level tablespoon

FRUIT (2 PER DAY)	1 SERVING EQUAL TO:
Banana	1 small
Berries e.g. blackberries, raspberries	1 cup (80 g/2 ½ oz)
Dried fruit	3 dried apricots/handful raisins
Fruit juice	Small glass (125 ml/4 fl oz)*
Grapes, cherries	15
Grapefruit	½ whole fruit
Large fruit e.g. melon, pineapple, papaya	1 slice
Medium fruit e.g. oranges, pear, apple	1 fruit
Small fruit e.g. clementine, plums	2 fruits
Any stewed fruit (unsweetened or with sweetener)	3 level tablespoons
Any tinned fruit (in natural juice)	3 level tablespoons

DRINKS	At least 8 drinks or 2 litres (4 pints) a day
Water (still or sparkling)	Unlimited
Tea and coffee, caffeinated or decaffeinated	Unlimited
Fruit, herbal or green teas	Unlimited
Sugar-free or diet squash or fizzy drinks	Up to a maximum of 9 cans (3 litres/6 pints) per week

ALCOHOL	UNITS	CALORIES
Up to max.10 units (100 g) alcohol per week.		
Wine 13% (250 ml/8½ oz)	3.3	240
Cider (568 ml/1 pint bottle)	2.3	210
Pint of beer/lager 4% (568 ml/1 pint)	2.3	170
Wine 13% (175 ml/6 fl oz)	2.3	170
Champagne (125 ml/4 fl oz)	1.5	100
Alcopop 5% (275 ml/9 fl oz bottle)	1.4	200
Port (50 ml/1¾ fl oz)	1	79
Sherry (50 ml/1¾ fl oz)	1	58
Gin and slimline tonic (25 ml/1 fl oz gin Δ)	1	50

Δ A standard pub measure not home-poured.

TREATS (UP TO 3 PER WEEK)	SERVINGS
Crisps*	1 small packet (25–30 g/3/4–1 oz)
Plain or chocolate biscuits (e.g. digestive)	2
Chocolate (ideally dark 70 per cent cocoa or higher content)	5 small squares or 30 g (1 oz)
Ice cream	2 scoops standard or 1 scoop luxury
Malt loaf	1 slice
Hot cross bun	1 bun
Fruity bread or teacake	1 teacake
Fairy cakes	2 small cakes with thin or no icing
Flapjack	2 'mini bites' (3 cm/1 in square)
Jaffa cakes, ginger nuts or small chocolate-chip cookies	3
Individual chocolate or truffle	3
Rich tea biscuits	4
Chocolate bar	½ a 58 g bar or a funsize bar
Cereal bar	1

Δ Limit to 1 glass of fruit and vegetable juice per day * Try to limit these salty foods to once during your five unrestricted days

ready reckoners for weight loss

MALE weight loss servings/up to 12½ stone (79 kg)

Use these tables to work out how many servings you can eat throughout the week according to your age, sex and current weight.

	2 RESTRICTED DAYS	5 UNRESTRICTED DAYS														
		Less than 8½ stone (54 kg)			8½–9½ stone (54–60 kg)			9½–10½ stone (60–67 kg)			10½–11½ stone (67–73 kg)			11½–12½ stone (73–79 kg)		
Age		18–29	30–60	60+	18–29	30–60	60+	18–29	30–60	60+	18–29	30–60	60+	18–29	30–60	60+
Maximum kcal per day	1,100	1,600	1,600	1,400	1,700	1,600	1,400	1,900	1,800	1,600	2,000	1,900	1,700	2,100	2,000	1,800
Carbohydrate servings	0	max 7	max 7	max 6	max 7	max 7	max 6	max 8	max 8	max 7	max 9	max 9	max 7	max 11	max 9	max 8
Protein servings	min 4 max 14	min 3 max 9	min 3 max 9	min 3 max 8	min 4 max 10	min 4 max 9	min 4 max 8	min 5 max 12	min 5 max 11	min 5 max 9	min 6 max 14	min 6 max 12	min 6 max 10	min 7 max 14	min 7 max 14	min 7 max 11
Fat servings	max 6	max 4	max 4	max 3	max 5	max 4	max 3	max 5	max 5	max 4	max 5	max 5	max 5	max 5	max 5	max 5
Dairy servings	3 (recommended)	3 (recommended for all weight groups)														
Vegetable servings	5 (recommended)	5 (recommended for all weight groups)														
Fruit servings	1 (recommended)	2 (recommended for all weight groups)														

MALE weight loss servings/over 12½ stone (79 kg)

	2 RESTRICTED DAYS	5 UNRESTRICTED DAYS											
		12½–13½ stone (79–86 kg)			13½–14½ stone (86–92 kg)			14½–15½ stone (92–98 kg)			above 15½ stone (98 kg)		
Age		18–29	30–60	60+	18–29	30–60	60+	18–29	30–60	60+	18–29	30–60	60+
Maximum kcal per day	1,100	2,300	2,200	2,000	2,500	2,300	2,100	2,500	2,400	2,200	2,500	2,500	2,300
Carbohydrate servings	0	max 12	max 11	max 9	max 13	max 12	max 11	max 13	max 12	max 11	max 13	max 13	max 12
Protein servings	min 4 max 14	min 8 max 16	min 8 max 15	min 8 max 14	min 9 max 17	min 9 max 16	min 9 max 14	min 10 max 17	min 10 max 17	min 10 max 15	min 11 max 17	min 11 max 17	min 11 max 16
Fat servings	max 6	max 6	max 5	max 5	max 7	max 6	max 5	max 7	max 6	max 5	max 7	max 7	max 6
Dairy servings	3 (recommended)	3 (recommended for all weight groups)											
Vegetable servings	5 (recommended)	5 (recommended for all weight groups)											
Fruit servings	1 (recommended)	2 (recommended for all weight groups)											

ready reckoners for weight loss

FEMALE weight loss servings/up to 12½ stone (79 kg)

	2 RESTRICTED DAYS	5 UNRESTRICTED DAYS														
		Less than 8½ stone (54 kg)			8½–9½ stone (54–60 kg)			9½–10½ stone (60–67 kg)			10½–11½ stone (67–73 kg)			11½–12½ stone (73–79 kg)		
Age		18–29	30–60	60+	18–29	30–60	60+	18–29	30–60	60+	18–29	30–60	60+	18–29	30–60	60+
Maximum kcal per day	1,000	1,500	1,400	1,400	1,500	1,400	1,400	1,700	1,500	1,400	1,800	1,600	1,500	1,900	1,700	1,600
Carbohydrate servings	0	max 6	max 6	max 6	max 6	max 6	max 6	max 7	max 6	max 6	max 8	max 7	max 6	max 9	max 7	max 7
Protein servings	min 4 max 12	min 3 max 8	min 3 max 8	min 3 max 8	min 4 max 8	min 4 max 8	min 4 max 8	min 5 max 10	min 5 max 8	min 5 max 8	min 6 max 11	min 6 max 9	min 6 max 8	min 7 max 12	min 7 max 10	min 7 max 9
Fat servings	max 5	max 4	max 4	max 3	max 4	max 3	max 3	max 5	max 4	max 3	max 5	max 4	max 4	max 5	max 5	max 4
Dairy servings	3 (recommended)	3 (recommended for all weight groups)														
Vegetable servings	5 (recommended)	5 (recommended for all weight groups)														
Fruit servings	1 (recommended)	2 (recommended for all weight groups)														

FEMALE weight loss servings/over 12½ stone (79 kg)

	2 RESTRICTED DAYS	5 UNRESTRICTED DAYS												
		12½–13½ stone (79–86 kg)			13½–14½ stone (86–92 kg)			14½–15½ stone (92–98 kg)			above 15½ stone (98 kg)		
Age		18–29	30–60	60+	18–29	30–60	60+	18–29	30–60	60+	18–29	30–60	60+
Maximum kcal per day	1,000	2,000	1,800	1,700	2,000	1,900	1,800	2,000	2,000	1,800	2,000	2,000	1,900
Carbohydrate servings	0	max 9	max 8	max 7	max 9	max 9	max 8	max 9	max 9	max 8	max 9	max 9	max 9
Protein servings	min 4 max 12	min 8 max 14	min 8 max 11	min 8 max 10	min 9 max 14	min 9 max 12	min 9 max 11	min 10 max 14	min 10 max 14	min 10 max 11	min 11 max 14	min 11 max 14	min 11 max 12
Fat servings	max 5	max 5	max 5	max 5	max 5	max 5	max 5	max 5	max 5	max 5	max 5	max 5	max 5
Dairy servings	3 (recommended)	3 (recommended for all weight groups)											
Vegetable servings	5 (recommended)	5 (recommended for all weight groups)											
Fruit servings	1 (recommended)	2 (recommended for all weight groups)											

ready reckoners for maintenance

MALE weight maintenance servings/up to 11½ stone (73 kg)

	1 RESTRICTED DAY	6 UNRESTRICTED DAYS											
		Less than 8½ stone (54 kg)			8½–9½ stone (54–60 kg)			9½–10½ stone (60–67 kg)			10½–11½ stone (67–73 kg)		
Age		18–29	30–60	60+	18–29	30–60	60+	18–29	30–60	60+	18–29	30–60	60+
Maximum kcal per day	1,100	1,900	1,800	1,600	2,000	1,900	1,700	2,100	2,000	1,800	2,300	2,200	2,000
Carbohydrate servings	0	max 8	max 8	max 7	max 9	max 9	max 7	max 11	max 9	max 8	max 12	max 11	max 9
Protein servings	min 4 max 14	min 3 max 12	min 3 max 11	min 3 max 9	min 4 max 14	min 4 max 12	min 4 max 10	min 5 max 14	min 5 max 14	min 5 max 11	min 6 max 16	min 6 max 15	min 6 max 14
Fat servings	max 6	max 5	max 5	max 4	max 5	max 5	max 5	max 5	max 5	max 5	max 6	max 5	max 5
Dairy servings	3 (recommended)	3 (recommended for all weight groups)											
Vegetable servings	5 (recommended)	5 (recommended for all weight groups)											
Fruit servings	1 (recommended)	2 (recommended for all weight groups)											

MALE weight maintenance servings/over 11½ stone (73 kg)

	1 RESTRICTED DAY	6 UNRESTRICTED DAYS											
		11½–12½ stone (73–79 kg)			12½–13½ stone (79–86 kg)			13½–14½ stone (86–92 kg)			above 14½ stone (92 kg)		
Age		18–29	30–60	60+	18–29	30–60	60+	18–29	30–60	60+	18–29	30–60	60+
Maximum kcal per day	1,100	2,400	2,300	2,100	2,500	2,400	2,200	2,500	2,500	2,300	2,500	2,500	2,500
Carbohydrate servings	0	max 12	max 12	max 11	max 13	max 12	max 11	max 13	max 13	max 12	max 13	max 13	max 13
Protein servings	min 4 max 14	min 7 max 17	min 7 max 16	min 7 max 14	min 8 max 17	min 8 max 17	min 8 max 15	min 9 max 17	min 9 max 17	min 9 max 16	min 10 max 17	min 10 max 17	min 10 max 17
Fat servings	max 6	max 6	max 6	max 5	max 7	max 6	max 5	max 7	max 7	max 6	max 7	max 7	max 7
Dairy servings	3 (recommended)	3 (recommended for all weight groups)											
Vegetable servings	5 (recommended)	5 (recommended for all weight groups)											
Fruit servings	1 (recommended)	2 (recommended for all weight groups)											

ready reckoners for maintenance

FEMALE weight maintenance servings/up to 11½ stone (73 kg)

	1 RESTRICTED DAY	6 UNRESTRICTED DAYS											
		Less than 8½ stone (54 kg)			8½–9½ stone (54–60 kg)			9½–10½ stone (60–67 kg)			10½–11½ stone (67–73 kg)		
Age		18–29	30–60	60+	18–29	30–60	60+	18–29	30–60	60+	18–29	30–60	60+
Maximum kcal per day	1,000	1,700	1,600	1,500	1,800	1,700	1,500	1,900	1,800	1,600	2,000	1,900	1,700
Carbohydrate servings	0	max 7	max 7	max 6	max 8	max 7	max 6	max 9	max 8	max 7	max 9	max 9	max 7
Protein servings	min 4 max 12	min 3 max 10	min 3 max 9	min 3 max 8	min 4 max 11	min 4 max 10	min 4 max 8	min 5 max 12	min 5 max 11	min 5 max 9	min 6 max 14	min 6 max 12	min 6 max 10
Fat servings	max 5	max 5	max 4	max 4	max 5	max 5	max 4	max 5	max 5	max 4	max 5	max 5	max 5
Dairy servings	3 (recommended)	3 (recommended for all weight groups)											
Vegetable servings	5 (recommended)	5 (recommended for all weight groups)											
Fruit servings	1 (recommended)	2 (recommended for all weight groups)											

FEMALE weight maintenance servings/over 11½ stone (73 kg)

	1 RESTRICTED DAY	6 UNRESTRICTED DAYS											
		11½–12½ stone (73–79 kg)			12½–13½ stone (79–86 kg)			13½–14½ stone (86–92 kg)			above 14½ stone (92 kg)		
Age		18–29	30–60	60+	18–29	30–60	60+	18–29	30–60	60+	18–29	30–60	60+
Maximum kcal per day	1,000	2,000	1,900	1,800	2,000	2,000	1,900	2,000	2,000	2,000	2,000	2,000	2,000
Carbohydrate servings	0	max 9	max 9	max 8	max 9	max 9	max 9	max 9	max 9	max 9	max 9	max 9	max 9
Protein servings	min 4 max 12	min 7 max 14	min 7 max 12	min 7 max 11	min 8 max 14	min 8 max 14	min 8 max 12	min 9 max 14	min 9 max 14	min 9 max 14	min 10 max 14	min 10 max 14	min 10 max 14
Fat servings	max 5	max 5	max 5	max 5	max 5	max 5	max 5	max 5	max 5	max 5	max 5	max 5	max 5
Dairy servings	3 (recommended)	3 (recommended for all weight groups)											
Vegetable servings	5 (recommended)	5 (recommended for all weight groups)											
Fruit servings	1 (recommended)	2 (recommended for all weight groups)											

meal planners

Here are some suggested meal plans to help guide you through the early weeks of The 2-Day Diet – until the 2-day pattern of eating becomes established. We've given you three weeks' of menu suggestions, with your restricted days falling on a Monday and Tuesday. This is because many of our Dieters chose these two days as their diet days. You can, of course, swap them around if other days work better for you. It is probably a good idea to try, as much as possible, to stick to the same two days each week, so that The 2-Day Diet becomes a habit. However, the beauty of the Diet is that you can move the days around to suit your weekly schedule – some people find it better to diet on days when they are busy, whereas others find it preferable to diet on quieter days.

This section includes both standard and vegetarian plans that combine easy-to-prepare recipes with quick, healthy meals. Use the meal planners in whatever way works best for you. Some Dieters find that sticking closely to suggested meal plans helps them to keep focused, especially at the beginning of The 2-Day Diet. For those who want a little more flexibility, the meal plans will provide a great starting point to mix and match meal ideas.

Drinks have not been included in these meal plans, but it is important to drink 2 litres (4 pints) per day. Two dairy portions have been included in each day and it is assumed that one additional dairy portion will be used in the form of milk in drinks such as tea and coffee throughout the day.

Check the Ready Reckoners (pages 146–9) and food quantity lists (pages 142–5) to determine the appropriate serving size for you.

WEEK ONE

MEAL	MONDAY restricted day	TUESDAY restricted day	WEDNESDAY	THURSDAY	FRIDAY	SATURDAY	SUNDAY
Breakfast	Smoked salmon & dill omelette	Low-fat Greek yoghurt + raspberries	Sugar-free muesli Banana	Porridge made with semi-skimmed milk & dried apricots	½ grapefruit Granary toast, olive-oil spread & low-sugar jam	2 slices grilled bacon, Grilled tomatoes & mushrooms + wholemeal toast	**Recipe (page 96)** Wholemeal banana & flaxseed pancakes
Mid-morning snack		Handful cashew nuts		2 plums		2 clementines	
Lunch	**Recipe (page 26)** Spring green soup + celery sticks with low-fat cream cheese & peanut butter	**Recipe (page 39)** Smoked mackerel, egg & watercress salad	**Recipe (page 28)** Spiced pumpkin, soup + granary roll with ham & mustard, low-fat spread & sliced tomato Fruit yoghurt	Baked beans + granary toast & low-fat spread	Tuna, low-fat mayonnaise & jacket potato Large salad	Egg & tomato salad, wholemeal roll with low-fat mayonnaise	Smoked salmon, avocado & mixed leaf salad Oatcakes & low-fat cream cheese
Mid-afternoon snack	Handful nuts	Cherry tomatoes	Pear	Handful nuts	25 g (1 oz) Edam + vegetable crudités	Slice melon	**Recipe (page 138)** Soda bread + low-fat spread
Evening meal	Stir-fry beef, broccoli & mushrooms	**Recipe (page 72)** Herb & mustard-crusted pork fillet	**Recipe (page 118)** Fish pie + steamed spinach & green beans	**Recipe (page 110)** Turkey, tarragon & mushroom pie + new potatoes & 3 servings steamed vegetables	**Recipe (page 56)** Chicken & spinach curry with raita + brown rice Slice mango	**Recipe (page 126)** Vegetarian cottage pie + 2 servings steamed vegetables **Recipe (page 134)** Mini banoffee pies	**Recipe (page 112)** One-pot chicken & veg + roast potatoes & steamed broccoli Blackberries, low-fat yoghurt, cinnamon toasted cashew nuts
Supper	Olives	Milky coffee	Rye crispbread & low-fat hummus	Carrot sticks & peanut butter	Handful walnuts	Low-fat hummus & crudités	Wholemeal crackers & Camembert

WEEK TWO

MEAL	MONDAY restricted day	TUESDAY restricted day	WEDNESDAY	THURSDAY	FRIDAY	SATURDAY	SUNDAY
Breakfast	**Recipe (page 16)** Boiled eggs with asparagus & ham soldiers	**Recipe (page 22)** Raspberry & strawberry yoghurt smoothie	Bowl of porridge with chopped banana & walnuts	½ grapefruit Bowl fruit & fibre cereal with milk	Wholemeal bagel, low-fat spread, low sugar marmalade Yoghurt	**Recipe (page 98)** Baked ham & egg in bread cup	**Recipe (page 20)** Grilled kipper with egg + granary toast
Mid-morning snack		Handful walnuts				Milky coffee	
Lunch	**Recipe (page 29)** Indonesian chicken soup + crudités & cottage cheese	**Recipe (page 39)** Smoked mackerel, egg & watercress salad Bowl salad leaves	Salmon & cucumber sandwich on wholemeal bread Pear	Jacket potato, baked beans & grated low-fat Cheddar	**Recipe (page 45)** Pesto turkey salad + wholemeal pasta Slice melon	**Recipe (page 30)** Saffron fish soup + wholemeal roll & low-fat cream cheese	**Recipe (page 107)** Quick mackerel & horseradish pâté with rye crispbread Orange
Mid-afternoon snack	Hummus & celery sticks	Mozzarella tomato & basil skewers	Handful dried pea snacks	2 clementines	Glass vegetable juice Handful cashews		
Evening meal	**Recipe (page 58)** Griddled tuna steak with pineapple salsa	**Recipe (page 50)** Open spiced turkey burgers with guacamole topping + large mixed salad	**Recipe (page 114)** Roasted cod + peas **Recipe (page 88)** Instant blackberry frozen yoghurt	**Recipe (page 70)** Lamb steaks + tomato salad	**Recipe (page 61)** Herb-stuffed trout + steamed spinach & broccoli Chopped mango & pineapple	**Recipe (page 83)** Soya bean burger, low-fat hummus, pitta + mixed salad **Recipe (page 132)** Loaf cake	**Recipe (page 120)** Pork & apples + Steamed broccoli & spinach **Recipe (page 91)** Rhubarb fool
Supper	Handful almonds Cup cocoa with sweeteners		Crudités & low-fat hummus	Handful plain popcorn	Rye crispbread Small piece Edam		Small handful seeds or nuts

WEEK THREE

MEAL	MONDAY restricted day	TUESDAY restricted day	WEDNESDAY	THURSDAY	FRIDAY	SATURDAY	SUNDAY
Breakfast	**Recipe (page 19)** Spiced tofu scramble	**Recipe (page 18)** Skinny English breakfast	Bowl sugar-free muesli Grated apple	Boiled egg + slice wholemeal toast, banana & peanut butter	Bowl porridge & dried fruit	Scrambled eggs Wholemeal toast & low-fat spread Grilled tomato	Grilled kipper Wholemeal toast & low-fat spread
Mid-morning snack	**Recipe (page 22)** Yoghurt smoothie		Milky coffee			Milky coffee	
Lunch	**Recipe (page 44)** Green bean, broccoli & chicken salad Handful cashews	**Recipe (page 26)** Spring green soup ½ pot cottage cheese	**Recipe (page 106)** Salmon salad Mixed-leaf salad Oatcakes	Low-fat hummus, rocket & tomato Wholemeal pitta Yoghurt	Baked potato & cottage cheese Mixed salad	**Recipe (page 28)** Spiced pumpkin soup Oatcakes & low-fat hummus	**Recipe (page 40)** Crab salad Wholemeal roll & low-fat spread
Mid-afternoon snack	Piece Edam	Crudités & low-fat hummus	Carrot sticks & peanut butter	Small piece feta & handful of olives	Crudités with guacamole & low-fat hummus	2 plums	Handful plain popcorn
Evening meal	**Recipe (page 60)** Lemon & garlic prawns Small mixed salad	**Recipe (page 66)** Chimichurri steak Yoghurt	**Recipe (page 52)** Grilled miso chicken Brown noodles **Recipe (page 138)** Soda bread & low-fat spread	**Recipe (page 62)** Mustard salmon Slice fresh pineapple	**Recipe (page 63)** Baked smoked haddock Strawberries	**Recipe (page 75)** Venison & blackberries Steamed kale/spring greens **Recipe (page 134)** Mini banoffee pies	**Recipe (page 54)** Stuffed tarragon chicken + 2 servings steamed vegetables **Recipe (page 90)** Melon mint & pineapple granita
Supper		Handful nuts	Handful dried fruit	Handful nuts	Handful nuts	Wholemeal crackers Piece Camembert	Crudités & low-fat cream cheese

WEEK ONE vegetarian

MEAL	MONDAY restricted day	TUESDAY restricted day	WEDNESDAY	THURSDAY	FRIDAY	SATURDAY	SUNDAY
Breakfast	Recipe (page 22) Yoghurt smoothie	Recipe (page 19) Spiced tofu scramble	Granary toast, olive spread & grilled vegetarian sausages	Bran flakes & milk	Porridge with mixed seeds & chopped prunes	Fruit & fibre cereal & milk	Recipe (page 96) Wholemeal banana & flaxseed pancakes
Mid-morning snack	Large slice pineapple	Handful cashews	Apple			Handful unsalted Brazil nuts	
Lunch	Recipe (page 26) Spring green soup Low-fat hummus & celery sticks	Adapted recipe (page 39) Eggs, asparagus, soya beans, mint & watercress salad Yoghurt	Roast tomato & basil soup + granary roll & low-fat hummus	Recipe (page 102) Herbed quinoa salad	Jacket potato, baked beans & low-fat Cheddar Plums	Adapted recipe (page 104) Egg noodle salad Mixed leaves	Hummus, chargrilled red pepper & aubergine on wholemeal pitta Yoghurt
Mid-afternoon snack	Spicy fried tofu strips	Small piece Edam	Recipe (page 132) Loaf cake	Handful unsalted peanuts	Carrot sticks	Olives	2 clementines
Evening meal	Recipe (page 84) Stuffed courgette Small side salad	Mushroom & spring onion frittata Avocado & tomato salad Recipe (page 88) Instant blackberry frozen yogurt	Adapted recipe (page 56) Tofu & spinach curry + brown rice Stewed rhubarb & custard (sweeteners as required)	Adapted recipe (page 110) Quorn, tarragon & mushroom pie + steamed broccoli Baked apple & sultanas	Adapted recipe (page 48) Piri Piri Quorn skewers + rocket, tomato & new potato salad Recipe (page 136) Bun & butter pudding	Recipe (page 124) Lemon-scented quinoa & spring veg risotto + side salad Fresh-fruit salad + reduced-fat evaporated milk	Recipe (page 126) Cottage pie + steamed green beans & carrots Recipe (page 134) Mini banoffee pies
Supper	Olives & handful unsalted peanuts		Oatcakes & low-fat cream cheese				Handful unsalted pistachio nuts

WEEK TWO vegetarian

MEAL	MONDAY restricted day	TUESDAY restricted day	WEDNESDAY	THURSDAY	FRIDAY	SATURDAY	SUNDAY
Breakfast	Adapted recipe (page18) Veg English breakfast	Natural yoghurt with summer berries & crushed Brazil nuts	Wholemeal toast & peanut butter	Recipe (page 96) Wholemeal banana & flaxseed pancakes	Wholemeal toast, low-fat spread & low-sugar marmalade	Adapted recipe (page 98) Baked egg/cream cheese	Bran-based cereal with linseeds & milk
Mid-morning snack		Boiled egg Chunk of cucumber	Apple	Handful unsalted Brazil nuts			
Lunch	Recipe (page 36) Halloumi salad	Recipe (page 28) Spiced pumpkin soup + hummus & green pepper sticks	Mushroom soup Oatcakes & low-fat cream cheese	Sliced egg & tomato, low-fat mayonnaise on wholemeal roll Side salad	Adapted recipe (page 68) Thai tofu salad	Tomato & bean soup, chunk soda bread & olive spread Banana	Soft-boiled eggs & wholemeal-toast soldiers Glass vegetable juice
Mid-afternoon snack	¼ pot cottage cheese Handful walnuts	Olives	Grapes		Slice melon	Carrot & red pepper sticks, low-fat cream cheese	Handful unsalted mixed nuts
Evening meal	Recipe (page 83) Soya bean burger Yoghurt	Recipe (page 80) Okra & tomato curry	Recipe (page 126) Cottage Pie + steamed cauliflower & carrots Recipe (page 138) Soda bread & low-fat spread	Recipe (page 128) Bean & cheese quesadillas + ¼ avocado Strawberries & yoghurt	Vegetarian chilli with TVP & red kidney beans, toasted wholemeal pitta sticks + dollop of low-fat guacamole Recipe (page 134) Mini banoffee pies	Adapted recipe (page 116) Grilled teriyaki tofu + side salad	Recipe (page 124) Lemon-scented quinoa vegetable risotto Cucumber, tomato & basil salad Poached pears, fromage frais
Supper	Olives	Fried tofu strips	Handful cashews	Olives		Clementines	Fried tofu strips

WEEK THREE vegetarian

MEAL	MONDAY restricted day	TUESDAY restricted day	WEDNESDAY	THURSDAY	FRIDAY	SATURDAY	SUNDAY
Breakfast	**Adapted recipe (page 20)** Poached eggs, spring greens & chives	**Recipe (page 22)** Raspberry & strawberry yoghurt smoothie	Prunes Wholemeal toast, low-sugar jam & low-fat spread	½ grapefruit Granary toast, grilled vegetarian sausages + mushrooms fried in olive oil	**Recipe (page 96)** Wholemeal banana & flaxseed pancakes + blueberries & yoghurt	Porridge & chopped, dried apricots	Scrambled egg Granary toast + plum tomatoes
Mid-morning snack					Handful unsalted pistachio nuts	Cherry tomatoes Boiled egg	
Lunch	**Recipe (page 38)** Tofu & mushroom lettuce spring rolls Olives	Vegetable crudités, Edam & low-fat hummus	**Recipe (page 102)** **Herbed** Quinoa salad	**Adapted recipe (page 42)** Bang bang Quorn salad	Hummus, rocket & tomato sandwich Wholemeal roll + side salad	Baked beans on toast Raspberries & yoghurt	Tomato & red lentil soup Wholemeal crackers & cottage cheese Pineapple & melon fruit salad
Mid-afternoon snack	Handful unsalted mixed nuts	Boiled eggs	Apple Handful of nuts				
Evening meal	Tomato, herb & cheese omelette Side salad **Recipe (page 90)** Melon, mint & pineapple granita	**Recipe (page 78)** Middle-Eastern kale salad	Olives **Recipe (page 82)** Smoked aubergine salad + wholemeal pitta, yoghurt, cucumber & mint dip **Recipe (page 91)** Rhubarb fool	**Recipe (page 126)** Cottage pie + wilted cabbage & spinach **Recipe (page 136)** Bun & butter pudding	Chick pea & vegetable curry, Wholegrain basmati rice + yoghurt raita **Recipe (page 132)** Loaf cake	**Recipe (page 127)** Twice-baked cheese & leek potato soufflé Green & mixed bean salad	**Adapted recipe (page 63)** Baked smoked tofu **Recipe (page 138)** Soda bread & low-fat spread
Supper	Yoghurt	Celery sticks & peanut butter		Strawberries & yoghurt		Handful almonds	Guacamole & vegetable crudités

index

About the authors

Dr Michelle Harvie and Professor Tony Howell work at the Genesis Breast Cancer Prevention Centre, part of the University Hospital of South Manchester NHS Foundation Trust. Genesis Breast Cancer Prevention is the only cancer charity in the UK entirely dedicated to prevention. Because weight is a significant factor in the risk of developing breast cancer, Dr Harvie and Professor Howell have spent years researching and developing the optimum diet to help people lose weight quickly and easily as well as keep off weight lost in the longer term. This incredibly effective diet is the result of their clinical research. Dr Michelle Harvie is an award-winning research dietitian. For the last 17 years she has specialised in optimum diet and exercise strategies for weight loss and preventing breast cancer and its recurrence. Her findings have been published in many major scientific journals. She was awarded the British Dietetic Association Rose Simmond's Award for best published dietetic research in 2005, Manchester City Council's 2007 International Women's Day Award for Women in Science, and the National Association for the Study of Obesity Best Practice Award for best published obesity research in 2010. Professor Tony Howell is Professor of Medical Oncology at the University of Manchester. He has specialised in treating breast cancer for over 30 years and now focuses on pharmacological and lifestyle measures to prevent breast cancer. He is Research Director of Genesis Breast Cancer Prevention and has published over 600 scientific papers and book chapters, mainly concerning the biology of the breast and the treatment and prevention of breast cancer. All author proceeds from the sale of this book will go to Genesis Breast Cancer Prevention (Registered charity number 1109839) www.genesisuk.org.

Author's acknowledgements

Many thanks to Jo Godfrey Wood for editing the manuscript; Emily Jonzen for devising the recipes and Kath Sellers and Mary Pegington for analysing and collating the recipes for the book and to Debbie McMullan for her helpful suggestions. We thank the numerous dieters who have worked with us on the studies over the past 11 years, without whom none of the research would be possible, and inspired us to write this book.

Our greatest thanks are to Lester Barr, Pam Glass and the Genesis Breast Cancer Prevention trustees and staff who have consistently supported our dietary research for the past 11 years. Finally Susanna Abbott and Catherine Knight at Ebury for their patience and hard work in making this book.

Proofreader: Laura Herring
Indexer: Dorothy Frame